Get the Residency

ASHP's Guide to Residency Interviews and Preparation

Joshua Caballero, PharmD, BCPP
Associate Professor
Department of Pharmacy Practice
Nova Southeastern University College of Pharmacy
Fort Lauderdale, Florida

Kevin A. Clauson, PharmD
Associate Professor
Department of Pharmacy Practice
Nova Southeastern University College of Pharmacy
Fort Lauderdale, Florida

Sandra Benavides, PharmD
Associate Professor
Department of Pharmacy Practice
Nova Southeastern University College of Pharmacy
Fort Lauderdale, Florida

American Society of Health-System Pharmacists®
Bethesda, Maryland

Any correspondence regarding this publication should be sent to the publisher, American Society of Health-System Pharmacists, 7272 Wisconsin Avenue, Bethesda, MD 20814, attention: Special Publishing.

The information presented herein reflects the opinions of the contributors and advisors. It should not be interpreted as an official policy of ASHP or as an endorsement of any product.

Because of ongoing research and improvements in technology, the information and its applications contained in this text are constantly evolving and are subject to the professional judgment and interpretation of the practitioner due to the uniqueness of a clinical situation. The editors, contributors, and ASHP have made reasonable efforts to ensure the accuracy and appropriateness of the information presented in this document. However, any user of this information is advised that the editors, contributors, advisors, and ASHP are not responsible for the continued currency of the information, for any errors or omissions, and/or for any consequences arising from the use of the information in the document in any and all practice settings. Any reader of this document is cautioned that ASHP makes no representation, guarantee, or warranty, express or implied, as to the accuracy and appropriateness of the information contained in this document and specifically disclaims any liability to any party for the accuracy and/or completeness of the material or for any damages arising out of the use or non-use of any of the information contained in this document.

Director, Special Publishing: Jack Bruggeman
Acquisitions Editor: Robin Coleman
Editorial Project Manager: Ruth Bloom
Production Editor: Kristin Eckles
Design: David Wade

Library of Congress Cataloging-in-Publication Data

Caballero, Joshua.
 Get the residency : ASHP's guide to residency interviews and preparation / Joshua Caballero, Kevin A. Clauson, Sandra Benavides.
     p. ; cm.
 ASHP's guide to residency interviews and preparation
 Includes bibliographical references and index.
 ISBN 978-1-58528-365-1 (alk. paper)
 I. Clauson, Kevin A. II. Benavides, Sandra. III. American Society of Health-System Pharmacists. IV. Title. V. Title: ASHP's guide to residency interviews and preparation.
 [DNLM: 1. Education, Pharmacy, Graduate. 2. Internship, Nonmedical. 3. Interviews as Topic--methods. 4. Students, Pharmacy. 5. Vocational Guidance. QV 20]

 615.1071--dc23
                         2012023523

ISBN 978-1-58528-365-1

DEDICATIONS

Joshua Caballero, PharmD, BCPP

To my family, living and dead, who have always encouraged me to pursue my dreams no matter how far away they took me. To our pharmacy students, pursue your dreams no matter how far they take you. Finally, to my sons, may I support your dreams no matter how far away they take you.

Kevin A. Clauson, PharmD

To my parents Jim and Vicki for always supporting me, the most patient woman on the planet—my wife Angela, and the students who served as the inspiration for this book.

Sandra Benavides, PharmD

To my past, current, and future students for keeping me motivated, enthusiastic, and challenged. My hope is that I do the same for all of you.

TABLE OF CONTENTS

TABLE OF CONTENTS

If you have picked up this book, you probably know that residency applicants have about a 60% chance of securing a residency. In fact, the five-year trend shows the field getting even more crowded and competitive. We recognize the repercussions that it has in our students' lives, when after four arduous years of pharmacy school, they do not get a residency. So after watching some of our most talented and enthusiastic students fail to match, we developed an elective course for fourth professional year students to offer advice on navigating the tricky process of pursuing a residency and to maximize their interview skills. To our knowledge, this was the first course of its kind. But did it help our students? Well, over the past couple of years, over 81% of students completing our course have successfully obtained a residency or fellowship.

In the fall of 2011, with the vision of offering the proven benefits of our course far beyond the limits of our classroom, we began working with ASHP to distill our core advice into this slim book. In order to provide you, the pharmacy student, with the best resource available, we approached faculty and clinicians from across the country. These contributors have unparalleled (and first-hand) expertise with the residency application process and can offer insight into what residency program directors (RPDs) look for. We have also gone to great lengths to discuss related issues and opinions with RPDs from across the country to factor in differences due to age, geography, and culture. Through it all we made sure to require one characteristic from all our contributors— that they possess the same passion as we do for putting students in the best position to succeed. After all, you will be the ones to carry the torch after we are long gone. There is nothing superfluous in this book—it contains only the advice we consider essential, which has been effective for our students.

This book will bring to light many lessons that will make you a more attractive applicant to interviewers. The crucial details we share with you will be invaluable and help guide you on the path to successfully securing a residency or fellowship (starting as early as your first year). Be aware, you will encounter several resources and opinions that may conflict, but if you follow our advice and exercise sound situation-dependent judgment, you will put yourself in the best position to succeed.

One day we hope there will be enough pharmacy residencies and fellowships to accommodate all those who seek additional formalized training, making this book obsolete. However, until that time comes, we hope you take advantage of the tools in this book to maximize your skills and achieve your goal of getting a residency.

Joshua Caballero, PharmD, BCPP

Kevin A. Clauson, PharmD

Sandra Benavides, PharmD

August 2012

Editors and Contributors

Editors

Joshua Caballero, PharmD, BCPP
Associate Professor
Department of Pharmacy Practice
Nova Southeastern University College of Pharmacy
Fort Lauderdale, Florida

Kevin A. Clauson, PharmD
Associate Professor
Department of Pharmacy Practice
Nova Southeastern University College of Pharmacy
Fort Lauderdale, Florida

Sandra Benavides, PharmD
Associate Professor
Department of Pharmacy Practice
Nova Southeastern University College of Pharmacy
Fort Lauderdale, Florida

Contributors

Mary Amato, PharmD, MPH, BCPS
Associate Professor
Department of Pharmacy Practice
Massachusetts College of Pharmacy and Health Sciences–Boston
Boston, Massachusetts

Sandra Benavides, PharmD
Associate Professor
Department of Pharmacy Practice
Nova Southeastern University College of Pharmacy
Fort Lauderdale, Florida

Joshua Caballero, PharmD, BCPP
Associate Professor
Department of Pharmacy Practice
Nova Southeastern University College of Pharmacy
Fort Lauderdale, Florida

Editors and Contributors

Kevin A. Clauson, PharmD
Associate Professor
Department of Pharmacy Practice
Nova Southeastern University College of Pharmacy
Fort Lauderdale, Florida

Cathi Dennehy, PharmD
Health Sciences Professor of Clinical Pharmacy
Department of Clinical Pharmacy
University of California, San Francisco
School of Pharmacy
San Francisco, California

Shara Elrod, PharmD, BCACP
Assistant Professor
Department of Pharmacy Practice
Nova Southeastern University College of Pharmacy
Fort Lauderdale, Florida

Timothy P. Gauthier, PharmD, BCPS
Assistant Professor
Department of Pharmacy Practice
Nova Southeastern University College of Pharmacy
Fort Lauderdale, Florida

Deanne L. Hall, PharmD, BCACP
Associate Professor of Pharmacy and Therapeutics
Department of Pharmacy and Therapeutics
University of Pittsburgh School of Pharmacy
Pittsburgh, Pennsylvania

Jehan Marino, PharmD, BCPP
Neuroscience Medical Science Liaison
Field Medical Affairs
Otsuka America Pharmaceutical, Inc.
Princeton, New Jersey

Milap C. Nahata, PharmD, MS
Professor and Division Chair
Pharmacy Practice and Administration
The Ohio State University College of Pharmacy
Columbus, Ohio

EDITORS AND CONTRIBUTORS

Jose A. Rey, PharmD, MS, BCPP
Associate Professor
Department of Pharmaceutical Sciences
Nova Southeastern University College of Pharmacy
Fort Lauderdale, Florida

Matthew Seamon, PharmD, JD
Associate Professor
Department of Pharmacy Practice
Nova Southeastern University College of Pharmacy
Fort Lauderdale, Florida

Andrew C. Seger, PharmD
Senior Research Pharmacist
Division of General Internal Medicine and Primary Care
Brigham and Women's Hospital
Boston, Massachusetts

Laura B. Smith, PharmD, BCPS (AQ ID)
Clinical Pharmacist, Infectious Diseases
Department of Pharmacy
Jackson Memorial Hospital
Miami, Florida

Jennifer G. Steinberg, PharmD, BCPS
Assistant Professor
Department of Pharmacy Practice
Nova Southeastern University College of Pharmacy
Fort Lauderdale, Florida

Jessica Wine, PharmD
Staff Pharmacist
Department of Pharmacy
Baptist Hospital of Miami
Miami, Florida

CHAPTER I

Preparing to Compete for a Pharmacy Residency

Joshua Caballero, PharmD, BCPP
Kevin A. Clauson, PharmD
Sandra Benavides, PharmD

Many factors have contributed to the escalating level of competition for securing a pharmacy residency in the United States. These include an increasing number of students graduating from more pharmacy programs, declining job opportunities for new graduates in some regions, and interest in further training to be competitive for patient-focused or other specialized positions. The gap between the number of residency positions available and the number of positions needed to train all interested and qualified graduates is rapidly increasing every year. Thus, it is critical for you to prepare well for the residency interview process to maximize the probability of impressing residency program directors (RPDs), receive a high ranking, and ultimately match with your desired residency program. While some students decide that they will pursue residency training even before they begin pharmacy school, others do not make that determination until the ASHP Midyear Clinical Meeting (MCM) in their last year of school. Regardless of the year you decide to apply for a residency, there is plenty you can do to prepare yourself for this process. Although the focus of this book is on the interview and application process, in this first chapter, we will provide some guidance on how to prepare throughout your pharmacy school experience.

A Residency Is Definitely for Me (P1–P2 year)

If you decided that you wanted to seek a residency early on in your pharmacy education, during your first professional (P1) or second professional (P2) year or earlier, you will already have a head start on the majority of applicants. Not surprisingly, the core steps to developing your candidacy begins with grades. However, many other attributes such as leadership, teamwork, and publishing increase your chances at being successful in obtaining a residency. (See **Table 1-1**.)

Table 1-1. Plan of Attack: What to Do and When to Do It

1st Year	2nd Year	3rd Year	4th Year
First semester	**First semester**	**First semester**	**First semester**
Focus on academics	Focus on academics	Focus on academics	Work hard during your APPEs
Explore various organizations	Join one to two organizations (if not done P1 year)	Join one to two organizations (if not done P1-2 year)	**JUNE** Start writing your personal statement
Find out your faculty research interests	Seek research opportunity (if not done P1 year)	Seek research opportunity (if not done P2 year)	**AUGUST–SEPTEMBER** Update/finalize your CV (and portfolio if applicable)
Start developing and organizing your CV (and portfolio if applicable)	After finals, update your CV (and portfolio if applicable)	After finals, update your CV (and portfolio if applicable)	**SEPTEMBER–OCTOBER** Contact RPDs, and ask for letters of recommendation from preceptors, employers, mentors, etc
Save money for travel to residency/fellowship interviews	Save money for travel to residency/fellowship interviews	Continue to talk with upperclassmen about APPEs	Buy a suit (if current one does not fit)
		Begin making a list of qualities important to you and find programs you may be interested in applying to	Apply to the ASHP Residency Matching Program (if applicable)
		Save money for travel to residency/fellowship interviews	**DECEMBER** Attend ASHP MCM and PPS
			Finalize the list of programs you will be applying to
			Submit application materials to each program
Second semester	**Second semester**	**Second semester**	**Second semester**
Focus on academics	Focus on academics	Focus on academics	**JANUARY** Secure interviews
Consider joining one to two organizations	Maintain involvement in one to two organizations	Maintain involvement in one to two organizations	**FEBRUARY** Interview

Table 1-1. Plan of Attack: What to Do and When to Do It (cont'd)

1st Year	2nd Year	3rd Year	4th Year
Second semester	**Second semester**	**Second semester**	**Second semester**
Start talking to faculty to get research experience (either in the summer or in your second year)	Seek research opportunity (if not done first semester)	After you find out your APPE schedule, contact preceptors for the months of December, January, February, and March regarding the possibility of attending MCM and interviewing for positions	**MARCH** List your sites for the Match; Match Day; Scramble
Run for an officer position/head of a committee (this occurs near the end of the semester)	Run for an officer position/head of a committee (this occurs near the end of the semester)	Change APPE schedule if preceptor is not accommodating	Celebrate your success…
After finals, update your CV (and portfolio if applicable)	After finals, update your CV (and portfolio if applicable)	Save money for travel to residency/fellowship interviews	
Save money for travel to residency/fellowship interviews	Talk to upperclassmen about APPEs	After finals, update your CV (and portfolio if applicable)	
	Consider elective courses in your areas of interest		

APPE = advanced pharmacy practice experience; CV = curriculum vitae; MCM = Midyear Clinical Meeting; P1 = first professional; P2 = second professional; PPS = Personnel Placement Service; RPDs = residency program directors.

Study… Study… Study

Based on published literature and years of collective personal experiences, *grades do matter*.[1,2] The notion that "a C equals a PharmD" does not translate to the successful quest of securing a residency. During the first year, your focus should be on academics. For many of you, this may be the first time away from home and the first time taking such a heavy science load, and some of you may struggle with the academic rigors of pharmacy school. Although you can recover from an unfortunate beginning, there are ways to settle into the demands of pharmacy school and lay a solid academic groundwork for the upcoming years of education and your profession.

> From unpublished data, the minimum grade point average (GPA) needed to be competitive is around 3.3 and it may become higher as the competition continues to get more intense. Additionally, some residency program directors look specifically at clinical or therapeutic courses to see how you performed.

The first semester, in particular, can be distracting. You are constantly being bombarded with different organization events, rushing a professional fraternity, making new friends, and possibly exploring a new city. Make the time to have fun—but not at the expense of your schoolwork. Make sure you know how much time you have to devote to classes in order to be successful. Make learning, and not necessarily achieving the highest grade (although this is important as well), a priority.

> Watch your part-time hours; there will be plenty of time to work over the next 40–50 years.

Paying for a graduate education is stressful for many pharmacy students. However, if at all possible, hold off on getting a part-time job (or if you have one, decrease the number of hours you work). This is especially important if you know you require more time to grasp concepts. You will have plenty of opportunity to work (pretty much the rest of your life), and this time should be devoted to ensure you will get through the program. If you have a part-time job, it will almost definitely impact your grades and have little impact on making you a better residency applicant. *Let us repeat*, your grades are more important than your part-time job. Plus, consider the economic consequences of poor performance in a course. Falling a year behind due to failing a course not only costs you an additional year of tuition and fees, but also one year of a pharmacist's salary. Does a $250 paycheck every two weeks make up for it? Spend carefully so that you do not have to work, if possible. For those who must work, consider a job in a work-study program (where you may have more time to study), in a research laboratory, or in a pharmacy. It is never too early to begin thinking about forming positive relationships with supervisors, preceptors, mentors, and future colleagues. However, it is imperative that you allocate enough time to maintain a competitive grade point average. Being able to academically ace your first year will give you some cushion if you hold officer positions during your P2 and third professional (P3) years and your grades consequently suffer in pursuit of developing those complementary skills.

> **Your grades are more important than your part-time job.**

Get Involved in Professional Organizations

You will be inundated with opportunities to volunteer for a health fair, listen to guest speakers, and become involved in professional student organizations from the moment you set foot onto campus your first year. Pick events and organizations you attend cautiously. Take the first semester to explore what the various organizations have to offer. In pharmacy school, you may be exposed to well over a dozen professional groups. You most certainly will not have time to be a member of each and every organization. However, in your first semester, explore what the organizations are about. Go to the free lunch or dinners (you may be able to avoid purchasing a meal the entire first month of your pharmacy education), ask questions, volunteer for a health fair or two, but take your time to decide what organization fits your interests the best. Talk to the leaders and members in the organization to gauge how much time is devoted to the group. This will help you decide which organization (and leadership role) will best suit you in the upcoming years.

During the second semester of your P1 year or the beginning of your P2 year, commit to an organization. Joining an organization and holding an officer position is a highly desirable quality for an RPD. This will show the RPD that you have leadership skills, the ability to work in groups to accomplish tasks, and time-management skills. Remember… do not join every organization. Outside of the prestigious, invitation-only societies (e.g., Rho Chi, Phi Lambda Sigma), limit yourself to joining two other organizations. RPDs also want to see that you can remain focused. Joining one to two organizations and being an active member (e.g., holding an officer position, attending events) will develop the aforementioned skills that will assist you in successfully completing a residency. If you run for an office in an organization, be sure you are diligent in your work. This will also give you the opportunity to develop a rapport with your faculty advisor(s) and potentially secure that critical glowing letter of recommendation (also sometimes referred to as a letter of reference, or letter of support).

 Even though we encourage waiting a semester before joining an organization, an exception may be with pharmacy fraternities, which typically have students "rush" during the first semester of pharmacy school.

Get Involved in Research with a Faculty Member

In your P2 year, you most likely will have a good sense of how much time you need to devote to your studies. This year, you can consider taking on a leadership role in an organization (as suggested above), working with a faculty member on a research project or publication, increasing your hours at a part-time job, or volunteering at a unique pharmacy setting.

Consider working with a mentor on research. Research can take on many forms and does not always mean working in a laboratory. You may be able to assist faculty in a clinical trial or in a social and behavioral or pharmacy administration pharmacoeconomic study. In class, listen to what your professors are excited about and, most likely, that is what they are researching. Don't approach a professor just for the sake of being able to put "research project" on your curriculum vitae (CV); find a mentor you would like to emulate in your career and in whose research you have genuine interest. For example, if you received a Bachelor of Science in Psychology, find your faculty member that practices in psychiatry. If you have a passion for computers and informatics, perhaps one of your professors is doing cutting-edge research in that area. Faculty members are excited about sharing what they do with students and can often find a way to incorporate you into research projects. Most faculty members are in education because they have a passion for teaching, research, and service. As a student (in any year), you can contribute and assist faculty members by completing literature searches, developing and administering surveys, or working in a laboratory setting. The possibilities are endless. Oftentimes, a professor may have a stipend for you or offer the position as part of a research grant or work-study program, or you may receive elective course credit, which will serve a dual purpose for you.

 Pharmacy practice or clinical faculty primarily have clinical sites where they provide direct patient care. These faculty primarily teach in your therapeutics courses.

Research projects can result in a poster presentation at a national meeting or in a publication. Presenting research at a national conference is a wonderful opportunity to network with people from across the country. Additionally, we have heard of residency programs that only interview or rank applicants that have some type of publication on their CV. As such, you can approach a faculty and ask about writing a review on the use of a medication for a different indication (e.g., quetiapine for sleep; http://www.ncbi.nlm.nih.gov/pubmed/19299326) or treatment of rare conditions in special populations (e.g., acanthosis nigricans in children; http://www.ncbi.nlm.nih.gov/pubmed/18492785).[3,4] In the event that you have your own research idea, consider working with some classmates on something you find novel and important. I once had a couple of students approach me to provide feedback and insight into a survey they had developed on their own to conduct a small project. I was happy to read over the protocol, provide constructive criticism, and connect them with people that would assist in completing the project. Having an original and creative idea helps you stand out from your classmates. Keep in mind, however, becoming involved in research projects can be time-consuming. This may be the time you otherwise would have spent socializing with friends and family, or being involved in a professional organization. This time should not be taken away from your academic studies. Again, working intimately with a faculty member on research will allow the professor to get to know you and your abilities personally. If you do a great job, you may secure your second letter of recommendation. Also, here is something you seldom hear: *Most of us are genuinely interested in seeing you succeed and nothing gives us more pleasure in our career than seeing a student develop over four years and become successful in OUR profession. Seek us out!*

 You may find that some of the same professors who come across as intimidating in the classroom are actually approachable and encouraging when you seek them out one-on-one.

Start Developing and Organizing Your Curriculum Vitae

Every activity, officer position, and scholarly endeavor you attain should be placed in your CV. We recommend you update your CV every semester, if not every month. By staying up-to-date with your CV you will have less stress when the time comes to submitting your residency applications. It is very difficult to develop your CV when you are trying to remember what you have done over the past two to three years. Therefore, try to update it once every semester—possibly the weekend right after your finals are finished.

Clean Up Your Social Network

If you have a presence on social networking sites like Facebook®, Instagram®, or Twitter®, start cleaning them up! Better yet, be thoughtful about what you post on social networking sites to begin with, since you can only do so much to clean something up once it's out there. For example, even if you go back and delete some provocative things you tweeted, the U.S. Library of Congress is digitally archiving everything ever written on Twitter®, so you can never get rid of certain things. What you post may affect you as RPDs or hiring personnel may go to these sites to see who you are and what you do (http://www.ncbi.nlm.nih.gov/pubmed/20852165).[5] Even if you keep privacy settings as secure as possible, elements such as your primary profile picture may still be seen. Considering that social networking sites like Facebook® have been fined by the U.S. government over concerns about privacy, the implications of what you post may not be fully understood. Also, you may be "social friends" with a student who may gossip about your extracurricular activities to professors (believe us, it happens!). Worse yet, research conducted for Microsoft® shows that people conducting social media background checks don't always verify what they find there, so you might end up being penalized for something posted about you that isn't even true (http://www.microsoft.com/dataprivacyday). Every year, students across the country are likely failing to secure residency interviews because they have developed a negative reputation during pharmacy school. Pharmacy is a small world and sometimes information is relayed regarding your habits. On the flip side, this can also help you. Posting pictures of pharmacy-related events you have done may not win you any "cool" points, but it may solidify your attitude toward the profession in the eyes of an RPD. One tool you can use to rehabilitate, monitor, or build your online digital identity is Socioclean (http://www.socioclean.com). Readers of this book can redeem a free "social media report card" from Socioclean by using the code: GTRFREE.

 One approach experts recommend is to put everything you post on social media to the "boss test" first. If your boss at work saw what you wrote, or a picture you posted, or something you "liked," would it create a problem for you?

 Recognize that some pharmacy students gossip and this can affect your candidacy. Also, be aware that your picture may be taken and "tagged" without you even knowing it, so be careful of how you conduct yourself and be cognizant about monitoring your online presence.

 Try to capitalize on the professional networking opportunities that social media offers. One pharmacy student hosted a #scriptyourfuture chat on Twitter® about medication adherence that was so popular it became a trending topic and helped increase awareness on the subject. Another student was immortalized in a book about using social media to drive positive social change.

Explore Your Passions

By your P3 year, you are probably beginning to realize where your passions lie. You do not necessarily have to have them set in stone, but your exposure to introductory pharmacy practice experiences (IPPEs); professional organizations; and therapeutic/clinical course work or research may have sparked an interest in a particular field of pharmacy. It is a great idea to begin to network with faculty or preceptors that have sparked this interest. For example, a student who knows she wants to work in pediatrics may contact the pediatric pharmacist where she is assigned for an IPPE or the faculty member that practices in pediatrics to shadow and discuss postgraduate training and job opportunities. This is a great way to network and learn more about the field. Consider taking electives in areas you are interested in (e.g., women's health) to supplement your learning and to connect with the faculty. Be prepared in advance for these courses and engage with your professors. The smaller class size of electives allows your faculty to get to know you better, which may prove useful during your residency application process (again, another potential person to write a letter of recommendation for you).

Selecting Your APPEs

Your P3 year is an exciting year, particularly as you begin to choose your advanced pharmacy practice experiences (APPEs). Don't discount the importance of selecting APPEs. Talk with upperclassmen to determine which APPE was a challenging and positive experience. Don't shy away from rotations because the preceptor is "hard." Choose a variety of APPEs, and if possible, in a variety of locations. Having this diversity of rotations allows you to explore career options you may not have considered and reflects your adaptability. If you are considering applying to a residency program in your area, think about selecting a few APPEs at that site to get a first-hand experience at what the residents do on a day-to-day basis (and possibly get to know preceptors of the residency program). Residents often serve as preceptors on certain APPEs, so you can see what a day in the life of a resident is like. Remember, any person you interact with during your APPE may have an opinion of your application to the program, if you do apply. Consider your APPE as a 1–2 month-long interview, especially if the site has a residency position(s) available.

One thing to consider when scheduling your APPEs is the time necessary to interview for residencies. If you are considering attending the ASHP MCM in December, consider requesting this month off or contacting your assigned preceptor to ensure it will be okay for you to take the time off. Of course, you should offer to make up the missed time on weekends or with special assignments. The majority of your interviews will occur between the end of January and beginning of March. Therefore, as you finalize your APPEs for these months, make sure to e-mail the preceptors as soon as you receive your schedule (even if it's nine months in advance). Your e-mail should convey a professional tone (see Chapter 3: Contacting Residency and Fellowship Directors for general e-mail guidance), describing your anticipated application to residencies and asking for the requisite time off to travel and complete the interviews. Recognizing that your APPE preceptors should be supportive in encouraging your professional development in this manner, your absence will likely create logistical or even legal challenges for them. Hence, you need to make sure you extend the same professional courtesy by accommodating whatever is necessary to make up for lost time (e.g., working 10–12 hours a day or weekends) or productivity. If the preceptor for that month is inflexible and unsupportive, you need to follow proper channels to modify your schedule. Ask your administrator of experiential education to switch your APPE, politely outlining the reasons for your request. To make life easier for everyone, we highly recommend students also request the month of February off (if possible) so that you can take the opportunity to prepare for your interviews and not worry about missing too much time. As with many of our suggestions, the key is to try and put yourself in a position to succeed. Don't forget to remind your preceptor of your earlier request once you begin the APPE and discuss what you need to do to make up the lost time in order to achieve the objectives of that particular rotation.

Lastly, you may consider asking your preceptor in the month of March for the day off when the results of the Match are released (referred to as "Match Day"). The day tends to be emotional (both for those who match and more for those who do not) and you will most likely be distracted. Also, in the event that you do not match, you can immediately begin to e-mail and call RPDs as soon as the list of unmatched programs becomes available. Over the last two years, by 6:00 p.m. of Match Day, many RPDs of unmatched programs had received over 150 e-mails and over 100 voicemails from unmatched applicants.

APPEs: Your Final Chance to Shine

The start of your APPEs marks the beginning of the last year of your profes-sional program, and often, you hit the ground running. How are you going to stand apart from the other two to three students on rotation with you on a particular month? More importantly, how will you stand out from the other two to 20 students your preceptor interacts with on a yearly basis? If you want to distinguish yourself from other students (i.e., your competition) in this environment, go above and beyond what is asked of you and more important-ly, show a genuine interest in learning and providing patient care. If you are requested to come in at 6:00 a.m., be there at 5:00 a.m. If you are expected to stay until 6:00 p.m., stay later. Of course, if you are coming in early and leaving late, make sure it is to prepare yourself or to follow up on issues that came up that day. Complete all assignments in a timely manner and to the best of your ability. Accept constructive criticism and ask for ways you can become a better student and ultimately a better pharmacist. If you have questions, research the information yourself before asking your preceptor. This shows you have self-initiative and are a self-directed learner. Your goal is to show that you are willing to perform at the highest level and do more than what is asked. If you have completed your assignments, ask if there is more that you can do. Below is an example of a student–preceptor interaction:

The first day of my APPE, I lay out to the students what is required of the rotation: when to come in, expected time of completion, assignments (such as drug information questions and patient presentation), and any other miscellaneous activities for that month. Somehow, most students are surprised to see that their grade is a "C" at their midpoint evaluation. They ask, "Why do I have a C? I have done everything you have asked me to do." To which I reply, "Exactly. You have done what is asked, which is what I ask every student to do... which is average, which is 'C' work. In order for you to earn a grade of a 'B' or an 'A' you have to do more work than what is required; hence, above average or excellent. When you enter the real world, there will be 'requirements' that everyone would be expected to complete. If you complete them, you will be average, because EVERYONE would have completed them. In order for you to stand out, you will have to do more than what is asked."

With this story, realize that even though an APPE preceptor may lay out the expectations and that you may receive a high grade (because they don't want to deal with a difficult student or receive bad preceptor evaluations) it does not necessarily mean you will receive a strong letter of recommendation or be looked on favorably when you submit a residency application to them. Even though this information is directed to your APPEs, keep it in mind for your IPPEs as well.

Consider applying to or participating in APPE-track, preresidency, or advanced clinical experience programs, if offered by your university. Currently, the authors are only aware of a handful of programs in the country offering such opportunities (e.g., Medical University of South Carolina, Nova Southeastern University, University of North Carolina).[6] These APPE-track programs have a variety of designs and requirements, so you should analyze the specific opportunities carefully before applying. Some programs are a complete year at one institution, while others may be only two rotations at one institution. Also, requirements may include any combination of the following: attending extra seminars, completing a drug utilization evaluation, finishing a clinical skills checklist, competing in clinical skills competitions, taking on extra electives, completing an additional APPE, and more. Many track programs are focused toward preparing students for a highly competitive pharmacy residency and/or future practice in a hospital or institutional setting. Note that such programs typically require significant efforts on the part of the students to acquire a certificate of completion. From personal communications, some applicants have been contacted or selected to interview primarily from their experience in such track programs.

DECIDING LATER ABOUT A RESIDENCY

If you are entering your P3 year or have begun your APPEs and realize you want to do a residency, there may be a lot of ground to cover in a limited amount of time. However, here are some things to consider:

- How are your grades? If they are not a solid B average, it will be difficult to compete. At this point, try to improve your grades by performing very well during the rest of your courses, especially the therapeutic sequences and stand out in a positive way during your APPEs.

■ Hopefully, you have been involved in organizations during your first two to three years and excelled in at least one officer position. If not, consider joining an organization if you are still a P3; however, note that it will be extremely difficult to secure an officer position since the voting usually takes place during the end of the academic year (April–May). Sometimes, there may be an opportunity to run for an officer position if someone resigned. But if you just joined the organization or were not an active member, it will be difficult to win the election. Despite this, you may still join the organization and be involved in committees within the organization (e.g., community outreach) and participate in their events (e.g., health screenings). Given all this, remember to join an organization that you like and have a genuine interest in. If you are in your last professional year, it will be nearly impossible to hold office or be involved in the events as you may have APPEs in different cities and spend much of your time completing all your APPE assignments. Remember to also consider professional organizations in your community, such as your local ASHP chapter. These organizations can provide opportunities to attend free, continuing education (CE) dinners and allow you to network with local pharmacists or RPDs. Often, you can volunteer to participate in a committee for such an organization.

A few years ago, Jamie, a pharmacy student in her P3 year, decided that she was interested in pursuing residency training. Her next step was to go to her faculty for guidance and recommendations. After discussing her interests and goals, Jamie narrowed her list of potential residency programs. Jamie was intrigued by one of the programs and took some unconventional steps to evaluate it. When she discovered that the RPD would be nearby to give a CE presentation, Jamie managed to make time to attend that meeting to observe the lecture—all while following proper channels at her school. The way Jamie executed this plan allowed her a rare face-to-face, extended opportunity to observe the RPD and see if he was someone she wanted to spend a year learning from. After the presentation, Jamie introduced herself and got to know the RPD. This was one of the most impressive efforts on the part of any student looking for a residency the RPD had ever encountered.

Jamie had already separated herself from other applicants before they had even started applying. The logistical effort of getting to the CE meeting just to introduce herself and assess the personality and teaching style of the RPD, and the support of the student's faculty enabling her to do so, all led to a very favorable impression of this student. Even without this extraordinary meeting with the RPD, Jamie was an excellent applicant. It was clear to the RPD that Jamie would excel in the training program, and he, of course, gave her the chance to prove it.

This anecdote reprises the unconventional efforts that one student took in evaluating a program and its RPD. For some, this example may blur the line between persistence and harassment, but the takeaway is that demonstrating creativity and a willingness to use unconventional (but sanctioned) methods to distinguish yourself may enhance your chances.

 During the ASHP Midyear Clinical Meeting, program directors sometimes give presentations. Take this opportunity to attend their lecture and see their teaching/delivery style. You don't have to approach them, but sitting in and listening to them may be a great way to gauge their program.

Now…A Little Bit About the Lingo

Now that you have decided to pursue some type of postgraduate training, you may be confused with all the acronyms and types of residencies. Keep in mind, the main purpose of a residency is to develop your clinical skills to prepare you for a career with direct patient care. There are two types of residencies: postgraduate year-1 (PGY-1) and postgraduate year-2 (PGY-2). A PGY-1 residency focuses on providing you with experiences in a variety of settings in order to obtain a general knowledge base. Some may have an emphasis on a particular area (e.g., pediatrics, ambulatory care), which allows for more time spent with a specific population; however, the goal is to provide rotations that focus on developing a clinician that can provide "evidence-based, patient-focused medication therapy management with multidisciplinary teams" (http://www.ashp.org/DocLibrary/Accreditation/ Starting-Residency/RTP-HowStartResidency Prgm.aspx), in a variety of patient populations.[7] A PGY-2 is a residency that builds on the foundation of the PGY-1 but focuses on a specialty area such as critical care, oncology, or psychiatry (http://www.ashp.org/DocLibrary/Accreditation/Starting-Residency/RTP-HowStartResidencyPrgm.aspx).[7] It is not a necessity to know what you want to specialize in when you apply for your first residency, but if you happen to know that you would like to practice in pediatrics, you may consider a PGY-1 in a pediatric institution or a PGY-1 that also has a PGY-2 in this specialty. When making decisions such as this, it is important to reach out to upperclassmen, alumni, past preceptors, and faculty to discuss your options. Again, many faculty would be happy to discuss your career development with you.

> **Programs with both postgraduate year-1 and postgraduate year-2 residencies may seek applicants who are interested in a two-year commitment at the same site.**

One question commonly asked by students is, "Should I consider a non-ASHP accredited residency?" The answer is complicated. Residencies that have obtained ASHP accreditation have gone through a rigorous process to ensure an optimal, auspicious learning environment for the resident in which specific educational outcomes are met. The ASHP accreditation process has specific requirements for qualifications of the RPD, preceptors, and the environment in which the residency will take place. All persons applying to a residency should review the ASHP Accreditation Standards to become familiar with these requirements (http:// www.ashp.org/DocLibrary/Accreditation/ASD-PGY1-Standard.aspx).[8] A nonaccredited program may be in *precandidate* status implying it has just started and is applying for ASHP accreditation. Or, you may also encounter a program that is well established and has decided to not pursue accreditation because they wish to be more flexible with how to structure the program, allowing for more personalization based on the resident's specific career goals and objectives. On the other hand, lack of accreditation or precandidate status could indicate the program is looking for "cheap labor" and offer a residency, which may not effectively prepare you. As you research the programs you are considering, be sure to discern which philosophy the program is employing as their basis for not seeking accreditation.

As far as PGY-2 programs are concerned, an accredited program can only take students who have completed a PGY-1, while nonaccredited PGY-2 programs can take any pharmacy graduate, with or without a PGY-1. Some PGY-2 programs may prefer to remain nonaccredited because they prefer having a larger applicant pool from which to secure a resident, or as mentioned previously, they feel they have a reputable, competitive program that has a track record for preparing pharmacists for successful careers in patient care. It will be your job to ask the right questions and carefully research these programs. Asking where former residents practice is a great way to gauge how the residency stacks up. Something to keep in mind is that if you complete an accredited residency, you will be able to apply for board certification soon after (zero to one year) whereas if you do a nonaccredited residency you will not be eligible to apply for board examination for three to four years.

 Board of Pharmacy Specialties provides a licensure examination that adds recognition to your degree and specialty (http://bpsweb.org).

The main purpose of a fellowship is to develop your research skills and prepare you for a career as an independent investigator.[9] There are mainly two types of fellowship categories recognized: traditional and industry.[10] Traditional fellowships are usually two years, primarily focus on research, include preparation for teaching, and are typically associated with a pharmacy program. The majority of traditional fellowships only take students who have completed one to two years of residency. Industry fellowships are usually one year (few two-year programs exist) and focus somewhat on research, but more so on providing the knowledge of the daily logistical operations of the company. The majority of industry fellowships offer positions to students who have recently graduated (i.e., completing a residency is not a requirement). While residencies are accredited by ASHP, fellowship programs can seek review by the American

College of Clinical Pharmacy (ACCP) Fellowship Review Committee (http://www.accp.com/resandfel/accreditation.aspx).[11] Because traditional and industry fellowships have radically different foci, it should be easy to determine which one fits your interests and career goals.

Finally, as you prepare and look for residencies or fellowships, it is very important to use sound judgment in talking with your classmates about which programs you are applying to. If you find a "hidden gem," be careful who you communicate this to. A "hidden gem" is a residency program you find that people are not aware of due to location, size, or recent establishment. You may have stumbled across a program during an Internet search or perhaps at a small booth tucked in a corner during the ASHP MCM. Whatever the case, nothing is worse than finding a program, telling your friends who are also looking for programs about it (perhaps even with the same interests that you have), and ultimately having 10 more people apply to the program.

I had a student who was looking for a PGY-1. During the ASHP MCM she found a newly established program that provided all the elements she wanted, including teaching opportunities, rotations in oncology and neurology, and location in a large city. In her excitement, she told her roommates who were also attending the ASHP MCM. This resulted in two of them finding the program as well and applying to the same program (even though one of them was not even interested in oncology/neurology but was happy that it was in a big city). The end result was disastrous. One of her roommates ended up matching with that program and she, despite interviewing there as well, was left unmatched (fortunately, she matched via the Scramble). The moral of the story is... be careful what you share!

PHARMACY ONLINE RESIDENCY CENTRALIZED APPLICATION SERVICE

Starting in the fall of 2012, candidates will be able to submit their residency applications using the Pharmacy Online Residency Centralized Application Service (PhORCAS). This is a web-based tool implemented by ASHP, which will streamline the application process for applicants, residency programs, and individuals writing reference letters. This will allow candidates to submit one application that will be disseminated to multiple ASHP-accredited pharmacy residency programs and allow for an easier application process. You can visit the ASHP website for additional information (http://www.ashp.org/DocLibrary/Accreditation/PhORCAS.aspx).

SUMMARY

The earlier you start preparing for your residency application, the more competitive you will be. As you can see, there are many ways to make yourself a viable applicant. Just as you prepared yourself in undergraduate school to gain acceptance into a pharmacy program (perhaps you even prepared yourself during high school to go to your undergraduate school of choice), you will have to take similar steps to secure postgraduate training. In the subsequent chapters, this book will focus on the application and interview process in the order the authors believe will provide you with the most direct guidance. However, you may need to review specific chapters as you encounter various situations. If you secured interviews and want to formally prepare, review Chapter 5: Formally Applying and Getting Ready for a Pharmacy Residency Interview. If you are working on your CV (as recommended) during your first year, review Chapter 2: Developing Your Curriculum Vitae and Personal Statement. Use this book as your guide in preparing yourself to secure that residency position.

> ## KEY LESSONS <

- Grades do matter.
- Reassess your need for a part-time job as your time to study or be involved in professional organizations will be limited.
- Get involved with organizations and research projects.
- Start organizing your curriculum vitae early and update regularly.
- Clean up your social networking sites such as Facebook® or Twitter®.
- Plan for your rotations and maximize their value and contacts.

REFERENCES

1. Mancuso CE, Paloucek FP. Understanding and preparing for pharmacy practice residency interviews. *Am J Health-Syst Pharm.* 2004;61(16):1686-1689.

2. Jungnickel PW. Grade-point averages and class rankings in evaluation of pharmacy residency applicants. *Am J Health-Syst Pharm.* 2010;67(18):1500, 1502.

3. Wine JN, Sanda C, Caballero J. Effects of quetiapine on sleep in nonpsychiatric and psychiatric conditions. *Ann Pharmacother.* 2009;43(4):707-713.

4. Romo A, Benavides S. Treatment options in insulin resistance obesity-related acanthosis nigricans. *Ann Pharmacother.* 2008;42(7):1090-1094.

5. Cain J, Scott DR, Smith K. Use of social media by residency program directors for resident selection. *Am J Health-Syst Pharm.* 2010;67(19):1635-1639.

6. New J, Garner S, Ragucci K, et al. An advanced clinical track within a doctor of pharmacy program. *Am J Pharm Educ.* 2012;76(3):43.

7. How to start a residency program. Available at http://www.ashp.org/DocLibrary/Accreditation /Starting-Residency/RTP-HowStartResidencyPrgm.aspx. Accessed May 14, 2012.

8. ASHP accreditations standard for postgraduate year one (PGY-1). Available at http://www.ashp.org/DocLibrary/Accreditation/ASD-PGY1-Standard.aspx. Accessed May 14, 2012.

9. American Society of Hospital Pharmacists. Definitions of pharmacy residencies and fellowships. *Am J Hosp Pharm.* 1987;44(5):1142-1144.

10. Melillo S, Gangadharan A, Johnson H, et al. Postdoctoral pharmacy industry fellowships: a descriptive analysis of programs and postgraduate positions. *Am J Health-Syst Pharm.* 2012;69(1):63-68.

11. About accreditation. Available at http://www.accp.com/resandfel/accreditation.aspx. Accessed May 14, 2012.

CHAPTER 2

DEVELOPING YOUR CURRICULUM VITAE AND PERSONAL STATEMENT

Cathi Dennehy, PharmD

Joshua Caballero, PharmD, BCPP

Your curriculum vitae (CV) is essentially a summary of your professional and academic career to date. Many residency program directors (RPDs) rely on it to deliver a snapshot of your accomplishments in order to formulate their initial opinions about you. Along with the CV, you will be asked to provide a personal statement (PS). Typically, the PS is intended for you to state your program interest, individualize the reasons for targeting their program, and describe how your strengths can be an asset to the institution. The PS provides an introduction of who you are and also allows an RPD to gauge your writing skills (e.g., can you write in complete sentences, use appropriate grammar, get your point across) and assess your judgment. The CV and PS (and supplemental materials when applicable) combine to form one of the key factors used to determine your eligibility for an interview. Therefore, this chapter will highlight how to make your CV and PS stand out in a positive manner.

> Some institutions require supplemental materials that involve essay responses related to specific questions about you or examples of past behaviors in a professional setting or career path. Similar to the personal statement, they are used to gauge your writing style and judgment.

CURRICULUM VITAE

Students commonly ask how their CV can be creative and distinctive. The simple answer is to be truthful and organized, while highlighting areas of significant involvement with professional and creative activities. The organi-zation and format of your CV should be easily readable and allow the reader to locate information quickly. When developing and updating your CV, it is important to explore various templates and styles. The student affairs office at your institution should have several examples to review. You may also solicit upperclassmen or pharmacists who serve as educators or clinicians to share their CV. Once you have an idea of how your CV will look stylistically, it is time to organize it. Organization and layout are key for ensuring a logical flow that enhances the reader's ability to process its contents.

Prior to assembling your CV, organize your accomplishments into categories by dates (see Appendix A: Preparing Your Curriculum Vitae: Format and Headings). If there are gaps in your educational or professional work experience timeline, consider addressing these in your PS. Below are recommendations that will provide you with a guide on having a polished CV that will impress.

Stylistic Tips

Create a CV with length suitable for your needs

One question often asked is, "How long should the CV be?" The answer: *as long as it needs to be*. Do not worry about your CV length: it is highly unlikely that your CV will be 15 pages long. CVs that include more versus less information about your roles and responsibilities in your advanced pharma-cy practice experiences (APPEs), professional activities, and scholarship activities are preferred. However, do not embellish your accomplishments. Most RPDs have seen countless CVs, and it is second nature for them to detect an artificially enhanced narrative. Again, there is no page limit to a CV. If the information you are including is pertinent to describing your character, commitment to your profession/public service, and professional accomplishments, then it belongs in your CV.

Use professional quality stock paper and appropriate color paper for printing your CV

White or an off-white/light tan/light gray, with or without a light watermark, is acceptable as long as it looks professional. Avoid lines, designs, or any-thing that distracts from the content. You want people to remember your CV for the content, not the color or background designs. Choosing to place the

CV into a separate folder/clear cover is a personal choice and is not re-quired—as long as the cover/clear folder is professional, go ahead. In the end, it is the content of the CV that matters and not the cover that it is in.

 Some decisions that students make will not be universally agreed upon by residency program directors (RPDs). As such, we feel RPDs will judge your curriculum vitae on content highlighting your accomplishments.

Avoid using fancy fonts

Font selection for your CV is a personal choice. For the purposes of read-ability it is fine to use sans-serif fonts or serif fonts as long as you are choosing a font that is easily legible. The style of the font you choose should also promote easy readability (e.g., Arial or Times New Roman) and not be too fancy (e.g., *Lucida handwriting,* ALGERIAN). The font used for subheadings should be boldfaced and of a conventional font size that is easily readable (14 pt) while all other text should be standard 12 pt.

Be consistent

All formatting should be consistent throughout your CV. CVs that have formatting changes from page to page (e.g., differences in font, indentation, heading style – some are underlined while others are set in boldface) reflect poorly on you. Failure to be consistent with formatting is analogous to a preventable medication error; each suggests a lack of attention to detail that can prove deleterious to a patient or to your candidacy.

 Proofread your curriculum vitae after you convert it to a portable document format (PDF). Page breaks and settings are often different than intended, especially when using free online programs.

Organizational Tips

Hopefully, you've been updating your CV regularly. However, if you are putting it together for the first time since you began pharmacy school, you have a lot of work to do (which is not a bad thing… that may just mean you have been busy). Remember to organize your activities into specific headings.

Appendix A: Preparing Your Curriculum Vitae: Format and Headings provides examples of common headings used for pharmacy CVs. However, below are additional tips to make sure your CV effectively conveys your work.

Clearly state your name and how you can be reached

Your name and contact information should be placed on the top of the first page. It should include a reliable address (mail and e-mail) and a phone that you can be easily reached at, such as your mobile phone.

If not using your pharmacy program's e-mail address, use a professional e-mail address (e.g., johnsmith@XYZ.com).

Provide explanations for items

All activities and acronyms in your CV should be clearly explained. You should not expect the reader to interpret these on their own, as in some cases they may be misinterpreted to mean something they are not. The person reviewing your CV may be a practicing pharmacist, an administrator far removed from clinical practice, or a representative from human resources. You should not assume that everyone knows what activities, terms, or acronyms mean.

Arrange items in reverse chronological order with most recent first

Having dates stand out in a column to the left with the activity stated to the right is one approach to cleanly represent the temporal progression of your activities and experiences. Too often, students will group accomplishments, one after the other and then state the time period within the text of the accomplishment, where it can get lost.

Describe APPE roles and responsibilities

The residency year is centered on cultivating clinical skills, organizing and managing patient data, multitasking, and communicating effectively. Therefore, these are all prime characteristics to highlight in your role descriptions for APPEs. With this in mind, more versus less information about your clinical roles and responsibilities is desirable. For past APPEs, provide four to five bullet points or a short narrative piece about the scope of your responsibilities underneath each APPE listed. Highlight characteristics that show a higher level of responsibility. You may want to address the following questions:

- How many patients did you follow daily?
- Did you round with the medical team/preceptor?
- How were your recommendations communicated?
- Did you write chart notes?
- Did you advise the team during rounds?
- Did you make recommendations to the primary preceptor who communicated these to the team during rounds?
- What other activities did you perform (e.g., daily vital signs, medication administration record [MAR] review, pharmacokinetic drug monitoring, medication reconciliation, patient discharge teaching/counseling/facilitation)?
- If your APPE was one in which you were not afforded much independence, how did you attempt to create a more fulfilling role for yourself by reaching out to your preceptor, patients, and team to provide a greater level of service?

 It demonstrates a great deal of character if you find yourself on a rotation with negligible patient and team interaction, but you step up, show self-initiative, and try to work within the existing system to provide additional valued pharmacist services (some of which may even be new to the service model).

If you have not chosen your APPEs yet, you should familiarize yourself with APPE responsibilities in advance of choosing or ranking them. For future APPEs, obtain a description of your role from the preceptor or your institution's experiential administrator and include this on the CV.

Highlight honors and awards

This is a section that sometimes gets missed. If you were a recipient of an honor or award during pharmacy school, make sure you have this section to highlight it. You go back to any academic awards you have received such as National Merit Scholarship or Dean's Award; however, an award for being an outstanding social coordinator for your undergraduate fraternity should be omitted.

Include your professional work experience

Highlight any professional work experience while in pharmacy school. If you have experience as a research assistant or in a community pharmacy setting as a technician or intern, include it. Similar to the honors and awards section, including any involvement that extends into the undergraduate years pertinent to your professional roles and responsibilities as a future pharmacist, researcher, educator, leader, and involved public citizen, is appropriate. If you graduated from a particularly notable high school environment (e.g., Jesuit program, Charter/College preparatory school), you may include it since it may serve as a point of reference/discussion since the RPD may have come from a similar school and place an emphasis on it.

A commonly asked question is, "How far back and to what level of accomplishment should be included on the curriculum vitae?" The answer is simple: stick to professional activities or awards, such as working as a research assistant in a biology laboratory. Your work at a fast food restaurant should be left out.

Provide examples of leadership and professional activities judiciously

Most RPDs will seek out examples of involvement and leadership to evaluate you. However, do not misinterpret this to mean more is better. Due to increases in the number of applicants to residencies and number of available residencies, students mistakenly view the *quantity* of involvement as being more relevant than the *quality* of involvement. In reality, it will be much more valuable for the program to understand your motivations to become involved with any particular organization. Therefore, if you have been with five professional organizations over the course of your PharmD curriculum, but your level of involvement or roles are unclear or poorly defined, it will appear less meaningful than if you were involved in two professional organizations in which you were genuinely interested and took on a major role (e.g., officer position, organizing chair). Since your time as a student is finite, you should prioritize activities where your interest is genuine.

Feature types of presentations separately

Why separate them? In general, we believe most RPDs place a higher value on presentations and posters given at a professional meeting than on those presented on a rotation. Therefore, presentations should have their own heading. Presentations given as part of an introductory pharmacy practice experience (IPPE) or APPE should be separated out under a subheading (e.g., IPPE and APPE Presentations). If you have presentations or posters that were not completed during an IPPE or APPE, they should be separated under their own subheading (e.g., Professional Meeting Presentations and Posters). For posters, include each author's name (last name and first initials) in the order of authorship. Be sure you boldface your name so that it is evident that you contributed to the poster. This also helps the reader quickly identify your place in the project; a touch always appreciated by those evaluating your CV. Additionally, consider highlighting your contribution by listing one or two bullet points immediately beneath the poster. If authorship was listed by alphabetical order, a bullet stating this may be justified.

The appropriate way to list a professional poster is to include authorship; title of the poster (not capitalizing all the words in the title); name of the meeting at which it was presented; the city and state the meeting was held; and the month and year of the presentation. Appendix A: Preparing Your Curriculum Vitae: Format and Headings has an example of such presentations.

 If you had a name change during your education, setting your name in boldface type is a good way to indicate that this is you.

Be careful when listing publications

Many professional poster presentations at professional meetings will have the corresponding abstract published in the organization's journal. Some, however, are not. If you have a poster that also resulted in an abstract publication, list this as a poster on the CV as described above. If you have a published abstract affiliated with a poster, it may be included under a

Publications heading; however, state so with brackets at the end of the citation (e.g., [abstract]).

PORTFOLIO (OPTIONAL)

A portfolio is a binder in which you organize a professional copy of all your pertinent presentations, drug monographs, or journal clubs (e.g., given during APPEs), posters, or any other activities during pharmacy school you may be particularly proud of. Some pharmacy programs require that you create a portfolio and update it periodically. Even though it is not a requirement for most programs, some students make one and take it with them to the ASHP Midyear Clinical Meeting (MCM) to share during Personnel Placement Service (PPS) or to their on-site interviews. The purpose of the portfolio is for RPDs (and anyone else interviewing you) to view your work and see what you've done throughout pharmacy school. Additionally, portfolios can also be constructed online (often via software provided by the pharmacy program) and may be shared with RPDs or other relevant personnel in a more flexible manner.

Please remember that similar to your curriculum vitae, anything in your portfolio is fair game during the interview process.

PERSONAL STATEMENT

Do not underestimate the value of the PS. The PS is what gives RPDs a hint of your writing style: basically, it lets them know if your written communication skills are a strength or a weakness. Therefore, a poor PS can doom your application. Generally, we encourage students to remember that the PS is not a creative writing assignment but is intended to show that you can explain yourself clearly, use correct grammar and punctuation, and relay a clear message that answers the essay question(s) being asked. With Pharmacy Online Residency Centralized Application Service (PhORCAS), you will have the opportunity to personalize and upload your PS.

Do not forget that supplemental materials, such as essays to proposed questions, should also have proper grammar and punctuation and relay a clear message.

The PS format is similar to a standard business letter and should be printed on the same type of paper as your CV. Single-spacing is appropriate, and each letter should be addressed with the exact name and title of the individual who is hiring or the name of the RPD. Never send out a letter addressed to "Dear Sir" or "Dear Program Director." The general format of a PS is as follows:

- **First paragraph:** Introduce yourself and state the specific position you are seeking. State what your professional goals are; avoid being vague. Be specific regarding your goals and future plans. They may change over the course of your residency, but RPDs want to interview applicants who say they have *a plan* and "I hope to be ...."

- **Second paragraph:** Highlight the reasons the RPD or residency committee should consider you for the position. Address what you feel are your most important skills, attributes, or past experiences as they relate to the position you are applying for—do not restate your CV. If you are applying for a postgraduate year-2 (PGY-2) or fellowship position, you should state how this additional training will further your career interests and objectives. This could be a separate paragraph or included in paragraph two.

- **Third paragraph:** Bring closure to the letter and state what you will do or what you expect the RPD to do. For example, you could specify that you will wait for them to call and arrange an interview.

Additional Points to Keep in Mind

Avoid cutting and pasting your personal statement

The practice of recycling written work that you've prepared for one program for another program is not recommended as the question(s) being asked may differ, as will programmatic strengths. Every year, RPDs receive a subset of applications where candidates have mistakenly listed wrong institutions' names in their PS. This lack of attention to detail can make the difference in whether you are offered an interview or not.

Use proper grammar

Poor use of grammar is another preventable red flag that stands out in the PS. If you know in advance that you have some difficulties with verb tense or word choice, have your PS reviewed by a family member or friend and then proofed a few more times for accuracy prior to submitting your application. Also, some faculty may be happy to review your written assignments (e.g., PS, responses to essay questions) and offer suggestions. It is important to realize that faculty have multiple professional and personal responsibilities—do not take offense if they are not able to do this for you. If you are going to seek this type of intensive, focused help from your faculty, your best chance of success is to approach one you have an existing rapport with and give them ample time to review your work.

Highlight how program elements fit with your professional goals

How will completion of the residency program fit into your career path? If you really want to impress the RPD, you can also mention in the PS specific research being conducted at the institution you are applying to (e.g., "I talked to applicants from your program and here is what they said…" or "This impressed me as I'm looking for_____in a PGY-1 residency."). If the content of supplemental materials (e.g., essays) required by a program overlaps with some of the content of your PS, view it as an opportunity to include different elements in your PS that are not already discussed in your supplemental materials.

Avoid too much personal information

Personal information pertaining to age, relationship status, religion, and political beliefs should generally be avoided. Your PS and supplemental materials speak to your professional judgment. If you are communicating information that is too personal, an RPD may have some reservations. For example, if an essay question asks you to describe a personal or profession-al challenge and how you overcame it, it would be more appropriate to discuss a professional/academic challenge than to discuss challenges from personal relationships. In some cases, references to personal challenges can be introduced as part of an essay question, if this is the intent of the essay question. For example, if an applicant or family member has had experience with "lack of access to medicine or healthcare," this may relate to how you wish to shape pharmacy practice and improve access to medications. The key is to use this as an opportunity to focus on the professionalism you gained or maintained in spite of the personal challenge.

Keep it brief

Try to limit your PS/supplemental materials to one page. RPDs seek applicants who can convey their ideas and points succinctly. *Remember: attention to detail is key.*

Promote yourself, but avoid bragging

Your CV highlights all areas of involvement. If you are particularly proud of certain accomplishments, feature these (maybe the top two) in your PS. Keep in mind though that you are also trying to integrate how this program meets your personal goals and where this fits into your professional future. It is not about restating your CV.

Set yourself apart

Be yourself. Again, it is important that you do not view the PS as a creative writing assignment unless otherwise asked to do so. This is also true of any additional supplemental materials or essays. It is never a good thing to be too poetic or flowery in your writing style when it comes to a professional application. Alternatively, a PS that is too generalized is also not strong. Typically, these come from applicants who try to use a general or similar PS for several programs. Therefore, if you focus on your strengths and how that specific program can assist you in your future goals, it should be unique enough to stand out.

In conclusion, your CV and PS are features of your application that will determine whether you are invited to interview. Use this chapter's recommendations to put yourself in a position to get that invitation.

KEY LESSONS

- Keep your curriculum vitae organized using headings and maintain a reverse chronological order.

- Make sure that your curriculum vitae describes your activities and roles as bullet points as it pertains to research, leadership, advanced pharmacy practice experiences, work experience, and community service.

- Avoid using fancy fonts or paper colors that will distract from your curriculum vitae or personal statement.

- Personalize your personal statement and any supplemental materials by focusing on your strengths.

- Keep your personal statement to one page.

- Ask at least two people to review your curriculum vitae or personal statement for readability and clarity of content.

- Start early. Do not wait until a month before residency applications are due to start your curriculum vitae. If you add to it gradually over the course of your pharmacy school education, you are certain to have captured everything.

CHAPTER 3

CONTACTING RESIDENCY AND FELLOWSHIP DIRECTORS

Joshua Caballero, PharmD, BCPP

Kevin A. Clauson, PharmD

Sandra Benavides, PharmD

The first impression you make to potential employers will most likely be via e-mail communication. Therefore, it is crucial that you display effective, professional, and respectful communication when contacting residency or fellowship directors. This chapter will focus on these aspects to make sure the initial impression of you is favorable.

WHEN TO CONTACT

Contacting as a Pharmacy Student

One of the common questions students ask is when is it most appropriate to contact a residency program director (RPD). The short answer is, "As soon as possible." However, the answer is much more complex. Ideally, you should initially contact RPDs during late September or the start of October in your last professional year. Some argue to make an initial attempt to contact sooner, maybe as early as your second or third professional year. However, contacting RPDs earlier may not provide any advantage. Most RPDs have other responsibilities at their institution and might not remember all the students who *may be* applying in two to three years. Additionally, they will be focusing on the current year and sifting through a voluminous number of applications for their immediate positions. Unfortunately, many may simply not have the time to appropriately respond to a pharmacy student who may be considering applying "next year." Another issue to consider is that RPDs may change jobs or responsibilities and the contact you established (and the time commitment) may be wasted. Also, residency positions are sometimes lost (e.g., budget cuts) and therefore may not be available when you apply. Finally, your opinion may change about wanting to apply to a particular residency and may therefore place you in an uncomfortable situation if you have established contact stating a desire to apply, only to rescind that verbal commitment.

Contacting as a Current Resident

The exception to the suggested timeline is if you are currently in a post-graduate year-1 (PGY-1) and plan to contact a postgraduate year-2 (PGY-2) or fellowship director. Due to the specialized nature of that process and the smaller number of positions available, it can be advantageous in certain circumstances to establish contact prior to the September/October time-frame. This is especially relevant if the program has a PGY-1 position and offers a PGY-2 or fellowship. Moreover, if you know during your last year of pharmacy school that you plan to seek a specific type of PGY-2 (e.g., community, geriatric, informatics), this can affect your PGY-1 program targeting. So while common practice for contacting PGY-1 RPDs is September/October of your last professional year, the situation is a little more fluid when determining your timelines for PGY-2 or fellowship contacts.

How to Contact

When initially e-mailing RPDs, be direct and have an appropriate subject heading. RPDs may receive around 50 e-mails per day; therefore, your e-mail should be succinct and to the point. The heading should not be too long but have information that sparks interest. Headings such as "Interest in your PGY-1 residency," or "Applying to your PGY-1 residency position," are good choices. Headings such as "Residency," "Applying to your program," or "Residency questions" may not provide as strong of a prompt for RPDs to read them.

Your e-mail address should be your university assigned e-mail, but if you are using a different provider, please make sure you use an appropriate e-mail address. Addresses with words that can convey a lack of professionalism such as gigolo@gmail.com, fashionista44@hotmail.com, or rockyman@comcast.net should be avoided. Even addresses that you think are pharmacy-related and thus appropriate such as pharmacylove @aol.com, RockStarPharmD2Be@yahoo.com, and druggurl21@live.com can convey a lack of professionalism or judgment that may be off-putting for some RPDs. It is critical to remember that *your interview begins at the very first point of contact,* so you don't want to dig a hole for yourself with an unconventional e-mail address. Finally, make it a habit to attach your curriculum vitae (CV) and personal statement (PS) before writing the e-mail. This way you don't send the e-mail without the attachments.

Your e-mail should focus on the *5 Ws:* Who, What, Why, When, and Where. Let's compare examples A and B.

Example A

Dear Dr. Robbins, PharmD, BCPS:

Hi. My name is John Smith. I was looking over the residencies in big cities and found yours to be very interesting. I have a solid GPA and have been extremely involved. Attached is my personal statement and CV. Let me know if you have any additionnal questions and hope to hear from you soon.

Cheers,

John Smith, P4 stunent

Example B

Dear Jane Robbins, PharmD, BCPS:

Good morning. I am currently a fourth-year student seeking a residency for this upcoming year. I am looking for a PGY-1 residency with electives in pediatrics, psychiatry, and informatics. I identified the NY State Memorial Hospital residency position as one of particular interest as the experiences offered are consistent with those necessary to meet my professional goals. As requested on your website, attached are my CV and personal statement. Please let me know if you need additional information for my formal application submission. Thank you for your time and consideration.

Best regards,

John Smith, P4 student
President, Rho Chi
Nova Southeastern University

Never use the "Dr." and "PharmD" together such as "Dear Dr. Jane Robbins, PharmD, BCPS." It's one or the other, not both!

In Example A, John Smith addressed Dr. Robbins inappropriately by stating her doctorate degree twice (Dr. and then PharmD). The PharmD addresses the doctorate degree; therefore, there is no need for also using the "Dr." designation. There is no need to initially "toot your horn" by claiming you have a great grade point average (GPA) and been heavily involved. Your CV and PS can address those points, and they will be evident to anyone reviewing your CV. Also, stating you are interested because of location can signify that you are motivated by nonprofessional reasons. Other poor statements in this area include "I am interested in your residency because my boyfriend/wife/etc., live in the area..." It is important that you select a residency based on matching your talents and interest with a specific program. This will ensure that you have a favorable experience and be a productive resident.

The e-mail also has spelling errors (e.g., additionnal, stunent), which are unacceptable especially since there is a spell-check function in most e-mail providers. Also, double check the spelling of the residency director's name and do not ever address them by their first name; if the contact does not have a doctorate (e.g., PharmD, PhD), then use Mr./Mrs./Ms. as appropriate. Ending your e-mail with signoffs like "Cheers" may be considered by some to be too informal for an initial contact. It is best to consider using "Respectfully" or "Best regards." As you will often be uncertain of the individual's religious affiliations, caution is warranted in using references such as "In Christ" or any other derivation. When stating your affiliation/officer position after your name/signature at the end of an e-mail, do *not* include every officer position you have. Instead focus on the *one* that carries the most weight. For example, it's better to have a title for an organization's presidency instead of a secretarial one if you happen to serve in both capacities.

Finally, be cautious of any quotes in your signature section of your e-mail. Quoting nonexistent persons (yes, even Yoda) fails to convey professionalism or maturity. Overall, what does the quote convey about you that your CV or PS cannot... *nothing*! Therefore, the quote may cause more harm than good and may come across as pretentious.

Example B displays all aspects required of an e-mail: It states who (current fourth-year student), what (PGY-1 residency), why (areas of specialty interest), when (upcoming year), and where (NY State Memorial Hospital). It addresses the RPD appropriately, has no grammatical errors, and gets to the point. Also, the student placed his officer position and title.

> **Remember to save a copy of all your sent e-mails.**

Follow-up E-mails

Your decision about follow-up e-mails will largely be determined by the response you receive (or the lack thereof). Guidance in the form of examples is provided in the following section.

No Response

If you do not receive a response within 10 to 15 business days (perhaps shorter as it gets closer to the ASHP Midyear Clinical Meeting [MCM]), it is best to look for the original e-mail. Make sure it was addressed to the proper recipient's e-mail. If so, resend it with a simple follow-up message. See Example C.

Example C

Dear Dr. Robbins,

I recently sent an e-mail with my application materials for your PGY-1 residency position and wanted to confirm you had received it. Please see below.

Best regards,

John Smith, P4 student
President, Rho Chi
Nova Southeastern University

Note: Attach the e-mail you previously sent and re-attach any files, if necessary.

Still No Response

If you have not received a response after another 10 days, it is best to attempt to directly call the RPD. Perhaps the e-mail has not been delivered due to the server placing it in the "junk mail" folder, or the director had a family emergency (e.g., death in the family). If you get a voicemail, make sure to speak clearly and restate the 5 Ws. Always provide your phone number twice and at a slower than normal pace. Use a landline if possible, as calling from a mobile phone may be susceptible to bad reception and the message may not be clearly delivered. Restate your name and deliberately speak your contact number at the end of the message for the second instance. This prevents the RPD from having to go back and listen to the entire message again to get your name and number. Little time savers like this can really add up for a busy RPD overseeing dozens of inquiries. On numerous occasions, students have contacted us and failed to clearly provide their contact information, which prevents us from returning their calls. Of note, make sure your voicemail greeting is professional. Calling a student back and listening to an inappropriate voicemail greeting is a major red flag. A direct voicemail such as "You have reached John Smith's voicemail. Please leave a message and I'll return your call as soon as possible" is appropriate. Other considerations include factoring in if you have an accent, especially if it gets more pronounced when you are nervous, tired, or excited. If you are from a part of the United States associated with a prominent accent or from outside the United States, you will want to take extra effort to use a careful, measured pace to enhance clarity. Consider listening to your voicemail message to make sure it is clear.

Response

When responding, always thank them for returning your e-mail and then provide any additional information they request. Again, keep it simple and to the point as shown in Example D.

Example D

Dear Dr. Robbins,

Thank you very much for the quick response. Attached are the additional documents you requested. I will be at the ASHP Midyear Clinical Meeting and am registered for Personnel Placement Service. I am available on Monday and Tuesday between 9:00 a.m. and 12:00 p.m. I am looking forward to meeting you and further discussing the position.

Best regards,

John Smith, P4 student
President, Rho Chi
Nova Southeastern University

Sending the Wrong Information

Some of you, in excitement or haste, will e-mail the wrong attachments to the RPD. For example, you may send an e-mail with the wrong institution's name in the heading or send an unfinished draft of your PS. If you realize you made a mistake, take ownership. The damage might be irreparable. However, by taking ownership you may have an RPD that appreciates a residency applicant who takes accountability for his error and may still consider you for an interview. Again, the e-mail should be short and to the point. See Example E.

Example E

Dear Dr. Robbins,

I realized I sent you the wrong personal statement. Attached, please find the corrected version. I am sorry for any inconvenience.

Sincerely,

John Smith, P4 student
President, Rho Chi
Nova Southeastern University

Responding After an Interview

After interviewing, sending a follow-up e-mail to the RPD, as well as anyone else you had a significant interaction with is crucial (see Chapter 7: Following Up After the Interview). In the e-mail, thank the person for his or her time and input regarding the position. Additionally, address any questions(s) asked of you (that you were unable to answer at the time) to the specific person who asked the question. If Dr. Lopez asked a question you did not know, this would be the time to reply with the answer.

One year, I interviewed four students for a residency position. During the interviews, I asked questions that some of the applicants were unable to answer. After the interview, one particular student specifically asked me for a business card. The student e-mailed me within two days of the interview with a detailed answer (not a copy and paste from Lexi-Drugs™ or, even worse, Wikipedia) to address a question she had answered incorrectly. When evaluating applicants, this student stood out, because she went out of her way to answer a question asked of an interviewer who was not even the RPD. And yes, this person was offered the position and went on to be very successful. Moral of the story: It's the little things in life that sometimes make or break you. If you do not know the answer to something (and you are not expected to know everything), follow up!

 You are not expected to have the answer to every question. You can set yourself apart with a strong follow-up.

Personalize the e-mail when appropriate

If you met someone with similar interests (e.g., rock climbing) during the interview process, you should consider wishing them luck on their next trip. Also, address any of the aspects you liked about the residency (e.g., strong ambulatory setting). The line between being engaging and being obsequious is a fine one, so personalize—but be authentic. Finally, sending a personalized thank you note is a nice touch; however, an e-mail should typically suffice. (See Chapter 7: Following Up After the Interview.) Let's review Examples F and G.

Example F

Dr. Robbins,

Thank you for the opportunity to interview on Wednesday, February 15, 2012 for your PGY-2 specialty residency. I was impressed with your diabetes clinic and believe your residency will offer many opportunities that address challenges commonly encountered in your underserved patient population. Of note, in response to the question you asked during my interview, the most recent FDA guidelines recommend citalopram dosing should not exceed 40 mg due to an increase for irregular heart rhythm (prolong QT interval). I hope you have a safe camping trip in Montana.

Best regards,

John Smith, P4 student
President, Rho Chi
Nova Southeastern University

Example G

Dear Dr. Patel,

Thank you for taking the time to interview me on Wednesday, February 15, 2012 for your PGY-2 specialty residency. It was a pleasure discussing your practice site and the opportunity to engage with patients in your antiepileptic clinic. Have a good week.

Sincerely,

John Smith, P4 student
President, Rho Chi
Nova Southeastern University

Both these e-mails are appropriate and to the point. In example E, you addressed the 5 Ws: Who (John Smith), What (PGY-2 specialty residency and answered a follow-up question), Why (opportunity to provide direct patient care), When (Wednesday February 15, 2012), and Where (diabetes clinic). Example F is more direct but still carries the same message addressing the 5 Ws: Who (John Smith), What (PGY-2 specialty residency), Why (engaging with patients), When (Wednesday February 15, 2012), and Where (antiepileptic clinic).

Response of No Interest

If after an interview with a particular program (whether at Personnel Placement Service [PPS] or on-site), you do not wish to pursue the position, an e-mail simply stating this should be provided. The e-mail should be very short and to the point. See Example H.

Example H

Dear Dr. Robbins,

Thank you for the opportunity to interview. It was a pleasure meeting you and learning about your program. Unfortunately, at this time I am withdrawing my application from your institution.

Best regards,

John Smith, P4 student
President, Rho Chi
Nova Southeastern University

Overall, remember to maintain good communication skills during your e-mail or phone correspondence. Having good communication early on will set the tone for your interview and keep you on the road to securing a residency.

> KEY LESSONS <

- Use an e-mail account with an appropriate name.
- Address the program director and affiliated institution correctly.
- Use spell-check and ensure the spelling of the addressee's name is correct.
- Keep e-mails short and to the point while addressing the 5 Ws - *who, what, why, when,* and *where.*

- After a reasonable amount of time, do not hesitate to send a follow-up e-mail (or call) if you do not receive a response.

- Send a follow-up e-mail to everyone you interviewed with.

- If you did not know or could not recall the correct answer to a question during your interview, make sure to follow-up.

- Always keep a copy of all your sent and received e-mails.

- Be sincere…be yourself.

CHAPTER 4

ASHP MIDYEAR CLINICAL MEETING: RESIDENCY SHOWCASE AND PERSONNEL PLACEMENT SERVICE

Timothy P. Gauthier, PharmD, BCPS

Jennifer G. Steinberg, PharmD, BCPS

Laura B. Smith, PharmD, BCPS (AQ ID)

The ASHP Midyear Clinical Meeting (MCM) is held annually in early December. Nearly 20,000 pharmacists from around the country and internationally elect to attend this meeting every year.[1] Pharmacy stakeholders come for a multitude of purposes, and notably, the MCM serves as a forum for pharmacy students, residents, fellows, and practitioners to connect with potential employers. Job seekers and recruiting organizations place a high priority on finding the perfect fit for their needs, which provides an excellent environment for networking. Two major networking events at this meeting are the Residency Showcase and Personnel Placement Service (PPS).

The Residency Showcase provides a semi-formal venue for applicants to meet members of pharmacy residency and fellowship programs. Residency program directors (RPDs), current residents, and preceptors are typically present to meet, exchange information, and answer questions that assist applicants in exploring the pros and cons associated with each program. The Residency Showcase is an open session, which does not require appointments or registration. Alternatively, PPS provides a formal environment that should be considered equivalent to a preliminary interview, which requires both registration and appointments. The PPS sessions are more personal and time is devoted to you, the applicant, specifically. Residency and fellowship applicants may choose to participate in the Residency Showcase, PPS, or both. While attending the MCM provides many benefits, it may not be feasible or appropriate for everyone. You may consider not attending if you are:

- Interested in programs that are not attending the Residency Showcase or PPS.

- Limited to a specific part of the country and you have already met the RPDs via some event like a smaller local residency showcase, networking event such as a local professional meeting, or any other event (e.g., community health fairs) that may be offered by some pharmacy programs.

- Planning to only apply to places where you have completed an introductory pharmacy practice experience (IPPE), or advanced pharmacy practice experience (APPE), or have interacted with them in some other way.

Even if you decide not to attend, the principles discussed in this chapter can still be applied and assist you in successfully securing a residency. The criteria to review for selecting programs that fit your needs will be identical, but your method for obtaining information will rely more heavily on resources such as ASHP's Residency Directory; program-specific websites; direct contact with program representatives by telephone or e-mail; and communication with faculty, mentors, preceptors, and peers. Beyond this, your approach to the application and interview process will not differ from those that do attend the MCM.

TIPS FOR RESIDENCY SHOWCASE AND PERSONNEL PLACEMENT SERVICE

Although the Residency Showcase and PPS are different in their overall organization and function (see **Table 4-1**), several key aspects remain similar. Professionalism, preparation, gathering of information, and planning for the next step in your career are universal themes that encompass both venues. Following some practical tips will help you get the most out of your visit to the MCM.

Prior to attending both the Residency Showcase and PPS, you should establish specific criteria for your ideal position or program (see Appendix B: Factors to Consider When Evaluating Individual Programs). This makes navigating options at the MCM much more manageable and helps ensure you will select programs that fit your needs and ultimate career goals. Concentrate on these criteria when conducting your search and deciding

Table 4-1. Major Differences Between Residency Showcase and Personnel Placement Service

Residency Showcase	Personnel Placement Service
Semi-formal open sessions	Additional registration and payment
No additional registration needed	ASHP accredited and nonaccredited programs
ASHP accredited or accreditation seeking programs	Nonresidency positions and employers
More PGY-1 focused	More PGY-2/fellowship/position focused
Many applicants at once	CV posting
Each program attends one of three sessions	Online job search
	Meetings scheduled in advance
	One-on-one interviews (30 to 60 minutes)

CV = curriculum vitae; PGY-1 = postgraduate year-1; PGY-2 = postgraduate year-2.

which program representatives to talk to. It may be wise to initially explore a wide variety of programs such as those affiliated with an academic teaching center, a community hospital, a specialty hospital (e.g., pediatric hospital), and a government-affiliated institution. Residency applicants' experiences vary considerably, but you should expect to speak to 8–10 programs per day. Prepare questions in advance and know exactly what you hope to gain from speaking to specific program members (see Appendix F: Questions to Ask and Avoid When Interviewing, for potential questions). Consider topics such as flexibility in rotation opportunities, the amount of time preceptors spend with residents, or any area of specialized focus. Asking questions reflects genuine interest in the program and lets the residency representative or interviewer know you have your own personal goals to meet. Identify questions that are appropriate to ask the RPD or preceptor versus a current resident, and be sure to direct your questions to the appropriate audience. For example, the RPD will be knowledgeable about the schedule and reasoning for including specific experiences, while current residents will be more familiar with specific activities and projects performed during each rotation. Listen closely when speaking with the interviewer and try not to ask questions they may have already answered in your presence. Furthermore, do not ask questions that may be answered by reviewing the online residency directory (http:// accred.ashp.org/aps/pages/directory/residencyProgramSearch.aspx) or program-specific Internet sites. Such inquiries reflect poorly on applicants who have not done their due diligence prior to the meeting.

Examples of questions to avoid include the location of the program (although affiliations to specific hospitals or universities is appropriate), stipend amount, and other generic inquiries. Utilize the face-to-face time that you have at the Residency Showcase or PPS to ask those pressing questions that cannot be answered through other means, and focus on questions that can make or break your decision to apply to a residency program. During the MCM, take legible notes that will assist you in sifting through the information and organizing your thoughts after the meeting. Note that this is a guide and it will likely evolve throughout your search process.

    If a residency you are considering does not have a rotation in a particular area of interest, it is acceptable to ask if they offer off-site collaborative experiences with other nearby institutions.

Although the atmosphere at the MCM as a whole is business casual, your behavior and appearance at both the Residency Showcase and PPS should be reflective of how you would portray yourself in an interview setting. Professional dress is generally expected and business suits in conservative colors (may have a contrasting tie or ascot that complements the suit) are appropriate choices for both men and women. Do not mistake professional attire for dressy or trendy as there is a vast difference between a business appropriate suit and an outfit you might wear to a social gathering. Keep this in mind when choosing accessories as well. You do not want to be remembered because of your distracting tie pattern or oversized earrings. Furthermore, expect a large amount of walking and standing at both venues. You will be glad to have comfortable shoes and a water bottle. Chewing gum is discouraged. If possible, leave unnecessary items behind (e.g., backpacks, exhibitor items) as the halls can be crowded and you will have to maneuver through many people. If you do bring a bag, easy access to a pocket that can hold your curriculum vitae (CV), business cards, game plan for the day, and a map of the area can be beneficial.

    As you move about the Midyear Clinical Meeting, you will want to keep your hands free to properly greet people, provide your materials, and take notes.

Whether at the Residency Showcase or PPS always introduce yourself, offer your CV, and possibly exchange business cards with representatives from each program you interact with. This can be done when making introductions or before parting ways, but look for the prime opportunity when it presents itself to avoid an awkward exchange. Keeping all business cards you accumulate in one place can assist in preventing loss of important information. You may also wish to take advantage of one of several digital approaches to managing all the new business cards and contacts you acquire. The simplest way is to periodically stop to take individual photographs of each business card with your cell phone's camera. A more effective approach is to use an application (app) on your phone such as Evernote® (http://www.evernote.com) to manage the cards. In this case, you would similarly use the camera function of your phone to import the card image, and then you can tag the card, type a quick note to remind you of relevant details of your conversation. With this method, you no longer have to keep track of the multitude of physical cards you accumulate and you have access to the information everywhere you travel. Tools such as Evernote® often have handwriting recognition software integrated; in case you scrawled a note by hand on the back of a card and need to conduct a keyword search for it later. While Evernote® is a general information management app, there are other tools specifically created for this purpose including CardMunch (http://www.cardmunch.com). CardMunch is owned by LinkedIn® and can even auto-convert business cards into contacts for this professional networking site.

 Business cards may be useful for exchanging information when you do not have your curriculum vitae (CV) handy, but it is unnecessary to provide it with your CV as the information on the CV is sufficient.

As you talk with various programs and representatives, be respectful of people's time by arriving prepared and maintaining honesty when discussing your training, experiences, and interests. Make eye contact and be sure to speak clearly and in an appropriate tone. Be polite and ensure that you maintain professionalism even when waiting to speak with programs at the Residency Showcase or during the time between your scheduled interviews at PPS (for further details on interviewing, see Chapter 5: Formally Applying and Getting Ready for a Pharmacy Residency Interview and Chapter 6: Interview Day). Keep cellular phones on silent, avoid loud conversations, and be cognizant of your surroundings to avoid unnecessary distractions to those around you. Associating with other pharmacy students vying for residencies also requires you to maintain your professionalism.

Note that professional behavior extends far beyond the walls of the Residency Showcase and PPS. The profession of pharmacy is a tight-knit community, and it is important to maintain a good reputation. Plan to continue a professional demeanor throughout your entire stay, even after hours and when exploring the host city. The likelihood of encountering people involved in or recruiting for residencies outside of meeting sponsored programs is high when considering the large amount of people that attend the MCM. Also, be aware that many residency representatives have professional relationships with each other and it is common for them to exchange information regarding prospective applicants. You do not want after-hour activities to impact the impression you leave with the programs you are interested in, but at the same time, try to enjoy the city and do some exploring. Please note that while enjoying the city, keep your social network clean (see Chapter 1: Preparing to Compete for a Pharmacy Residency), especially if you are tagged in a picture or video.

Make sure to conduct yourself properly outside of the meeting, particularly at social events. Remember that there is a high possibility of encountering residency program directors and future preceptors in public.

During your search for a residency position at the MCM, it is important to stay calm and composed. It will undoubtedly be a stressful process as you attempt to plan your future career; however, it is an exciting time in your life, so try to enjoy it. These venues provide you the chance to put your best foot forward and gather information to make the best decisions for your future career plans. Keeping all of this in mind, preparation and a thoughtful approach to your activities while attending will be paramount to ensuring a successful experience at the MCM. **Table 4-2** lists some benefits and considerations to keep in mind when determining which event(s) to attend.

Table 4-2. Benefits and Considerations of Residency Showcase and
Personnel Placement Service Attendance

Benefits	Considerations
Many programs from across the country in one location can save you money	Travel and meeting registration costs
Face-to-face time with RPDs, preceptors, and current residents	Advance preparation of CV
Evaluate programs prior to submitting application/arranging for onsite interview	Large number of other applicants attending
Discover new programs	Professional demeanor at all times

CV = curriculum vitae; RPDs = residency program directors.

ASHP MCM Residency Showcase

The Residency Showcase, as part of the MCM, is the largest annual gathering of pharmacy residency programs and allows an applicant to meet with hundreds of programs from across the country in one location. In 2011, nearly 600 institutions recruited for over 1100 individual postgraduate pharmacy residency programs, with each program commonly supporting multiple postgraduate year-1 (PGY-1) or postgraduate year-2 (PGY-2) resident positions (http://www.ashp.org/Midyear2011/ResidencyShowcase/Residency-Program-Listing.aspx).[2] Participants include ASHP-accredited, preliminary accreditation status, applicant status, or preapplicant status programs and both PGY-1 and PGY-2 opportunities. Other types of postgraduate training opportunities (i.e., fellowships) do not usually participate in the Residency Showcase, although programs that include a variety of postgraduate positions may be willing to discuss other types of offerings during this time. In general, fellowships and nonaccredited residencies recruiting at the MCM are most likely to be available at PPS.

The Residency Showcase is included with your MCM registration and no additional fees are required. Information on meeting times, locations, and participating programs is provided along with other MCM information on ASHP's meeting website under the Residency Showcase tab and onsite at the MCM as well. The Residency Showcase is arranged into several sessions (approximately 2.5 hours each) to maximize the number of programs that can participate. Multiple programs participate in each session and are arranged in aisles of open-front booths similar to an exhibit hall (see Appendix D: Midyear Clinical Meeting Residency Showcase Floor Plan Example). Each program only attends one of the sessions and assignments are based on when they register for the Residency Showcase. As a result, there is generally no alphabetical or geographical organization to the layout and you may need to attend all of the Residency Showcase sessions to meet with all of your prospective programs.

The Residency Showcase can be an overwhelming experience due to pressures related to obtaining a position, the unique layout of the venue, and the number of attendees. To make the best use of your time and get the most out of attending the Residency Showcase, it is extremely important to have a strategy. Access information provided through the ASHP website (http://www.ashp.org/) well in advance of the meeting to map out a plan. Know what time programs are showcasing and where their booths will be located. Placing pertinent information in a chart or table is helpful for staying organized. The less time you spend trying to navigate the aisles finding your programs of interest, the more time you will have to meet with RPDs, preceptors, and current residents. Proper preparation will also minimize the potential of missing a program because you could not find them or because they were at a different session.

Any extra time left after speaking with the programs you have given priority to can be spent exploring the rest of the Residency Showcase, providing the opportunity to discover new programs. Take this into consideration and do not be afraid to approach a program that does not have a crowd. Programs may be recently accredited or be a last minute addition to the Residency Showcase, thus having limited advertisement. Such efforts broaden your horizons and you may be pleasantly surprised to find a hidden gem. As a rule, stay focused on your plan, but also be prepared to capitalize on unexpected opportunities as they arise.

Residency Showcase sessions are open and any meeting attendee with their badge may freely come and go from the Residency Showcase hall during times of operation, although applicants who are not actively seeking positions for the current year are asked to wait until the latter part of each session to enter. Applicants actively seeking positions who arrive early must wait until the session is open to enter the exhibit floor, which can lead to a mass of anxious applicants entering all at once. Note that proper planning, staying calm, not rushing, and being courteous will assist you in this environment. If you are a particularly anxious person, consider waiting until after the initial rush is over (maybe 5 minutes) before entering to avoid unnecessary distraction and pressure.

If you're not seeking a position for the current year, wait until the second half of each session to enter the Residency Showcase.

There are no appointments during the Residency Showcase and you are free to approach any program you like at any time during the session. You will likely want to meet with more than one program within each session, so divide your time accordingly and have a flexible plan of action. Expect to spend anywhere from 5 to 20 minutes with each program depending on the amount of information you are seeking and the number of other applicants at that particular booth. There is a thick and constant flow of applicants transitioning from program to program through the exhibit hall, which becomes reduced as the session progresses. Some programs inevitably receive more traffic than others and you may find yourself talking with RPDs, preceptors, and residents in small groups with other applicants rather than individually. Timing your entrance into groups should be done with care, so look for natural transitions as questions are answered and conversations end. In this setting, you may find it difficult to stand out from the crowd. However, professional behavior combined with a well-prepared CV and insightful questions will help leave a positive impression. When confronted with a busy booth, try to make eye contact with the representatives and become involved in the conversations. You will likely be excited and nervous, but it is important to wait your turn to ask a question. Many times applicants get flustered and forget their questions. Having written down your inquiry can help prevent this. Generally, booths are the busiest right after the doors open, as many applicants seek similar programs, which leads to overcrowding in certain areas of the venue. Booths closest to the entrance may be similarly busy immediately after the start of the session, so you may want to consider starting at the back of the hall and working your way toward the front. Consider doubling back to the booth at a later time if the programs you are interested in seem overcrowded. Keep on task and visit another booth in the meantime and give the busy area time to clear out. Near closing of the Residency Showcase times, booths tend to be less crowded.

Some Residency Showcase booths will be busy *all* the time. As such, feel free to speak with institution representatives in a group setting with other applicants.

With increasing numbers of attendees at the Residency Showcase, premium time with residency representatives is limited. It is of utmost importance to be prepared to make the most of your time. However, the Residency Showcase is not the only opportunity to have your questions answered. There is a vast amount of information available to prospective applicants through other outlets; therefore, it is best to do your research ahead of time and educate yourself about each program. Think of the Residency Showcase as a way to screen potential programs for a fit with your professional goals, expectations, and personality. Know in advance what you hope to gain from speaking with each program. Do not expect to leave the Residency Showcase knowing everything you could ever want to know about each program, but you should have a better idea of the program overall and of your desire to submit a full application and potentially travel for an on-site interview.

An important advantage of the Residency Showcase is the opportunity to see the current residents, preceptors, and RPDs in action. How they interact with potential applicants and each other can provide important insight into the dynamics of the program. Does the resident appear pleased with their decision to choose that particular residency program? Are they enthusiastic and do they take pride in discussing the program? Are the RPD and preceptors approachable and willing to answer your questions? Nonverbal cues are an important additional tool to help you distinguish between programs and gain an accurate impression.

The Residency Showcase is a valuable resource to explore the various opportunities available to potential applicants. With proper preparation and efficient use of time while in attendance, you can leave with a clearer understanding of your options and a better defined plan for your continued pursuit of a residency.

ASHP MCM Personnel Placement Service

PPS is a recruiting service that provides residency and fellowship seekers the opportunity to evaluate programs in a structured environment. In 2011, nearly 1500 pharmacy positions were listed at PPS and over 1700 applicants participated in the event (http://www.careerpharm.com/).[3] ASHP-accredited and nonaccredited PGY-1, PGY-2, and fellowship programs conduct interviews at PPS. Additionally, PPS serves as a recruitment source for clinical, faculty, research, and industry pharmacist positions. Institutions are represented from across the nation and internationally, allowing for numerous networking and interview opportunities without the added expense and time requirements of on-site interviews.

The intention of PPS from the perspective of an applicant is to provide an opportunity for you to personally meet with prospective employers and determine if their program can help you meet your career goals. At the same time, RPDs and department directors are searching for their ideal applicant. Each 30- or 60-minute PPS session allows for evaluation of your goals, experience, and abilities in comparison to those of the potential position(s). For those seeking residencies, PGY-2 programs are the primary focus during PPS, although not all PGY-2 programs participate. Alternately, the Residency Showcase is the chief recruiting ground for PGY-1 programs. This is mainly due to the large pool of PGY-1 applicants. As current PGY-1 residents look toward PGY-2 positions, the number of applicants to each PGY-2 program is typically much smaller and participation within PPS becomes more practical. It is not generally recommended to participate in PPS when seeking an accredited PGY-1 residency; however, it is highly encouraged for other positions.

If you decide to participate in PPS, you must register through ASHP's CareerPharm® website (http://www.careerpharm.com). Registration opens mid-September and allows you to post a CV and information online about your specialty areas of interest. Early registration is less expensive and posting your information early-on allows employers to find and view your information sooner. The search functionality begins in late October and runs through and after the MCM. Employers will likely view the site early and begin to set up interviews. Simultaneously, you are able to search for positions and contact program personnel. As stated in Chapter 1: Preparing to Compete for a Pharmacy Residency, you can begin to contact RPDs in late October or the beginning of November. The PPS website can be a bit overwhelming, as an abundance of excellent positions are available. Therefore, it is wise to determine elements of a program that are important to you before performing a search. Consider which rotations are available and if experienced and talented preceptors exist in your area of interest. For a PGY-1 residency, maintaining a general learning experience is important; however, the program should offer strong rotations in *your* area of interest. For PGY-2 residencies, diversity of experiences continues to be important, but if the program does not offer what is imperative to you, do not schedule an interview.

One of the benefits of participating in PPS is the ability to meet with potential employers face-to-face on neutral ground. Interviews are usually conducted by the pharmacy department director or RPD; however, current residents or preceptors may assist. Interviewers provide an overview of what the program has to offer, required and elective rotations, research projects, and responsibilities of the resident. Following this description, you will be provided a chance to ask questions to ensure you understand the position requirements and investigate opportunities pertinent to your specific interests. You should be prepared to answer interview questions at this time including any pertinent to your CV. It is not unusual to be asked about a topic from your CV (e.g., HIV/AIDS guidelines if you did a drug monograph on an anti-retroviral). Additionally, you should be generally aware of key issues in your stated area of interest and able to demonstrate how you have translated that interest into action. For example, if you state during your PPS interview you enjoy and have a passion for pediatrics, don't be surprised if you get asked, "So, can you tell me a recent article you read regarding pediatrics?" While you may not be asked granular-level questions during PPS, it obviously behooves you to be prepared for them.

 You should be prepared to answer interview questions during a Personnel Placement Service interview including any pertinent to your curriculum vitae.

Mancuso et al. provides an excellent resource for questions commonly asked to residency applicants (see Appendix C: Potential Questions Asked During Residency Interviews).[4] This article is geared toward PGY-1 pharmacy practice residencies; however, most questions are still pertinent to PGY-2 and fellowship positions. You should be aware of such questions and have already formed answers prior to arrival at PPS to avoid getting caught off-guard. Furthermore, answering these questions can assist you in further developing a vision of your ideal position.

Only registered employers and interviewees donning the required badge will be allowed to enter the PPS area. Your badge will be provided when you arrive at the beginning of the MCM. Keep this badge with you at all times during the meeting and do not lose it. When you arrive at PPS, be sure to have extra copies of your CV; however, most interviewers will have printed a copy prior to the meeting. Bring your interview schedule, including booth numbers, program name(s), contact person name(s), and other pertinent information. Arriving early and doing a walk-through can help you get an idea of the floor plan, which is quite expansive (see Appendix E: Midyear Clinical Meeting Personnel Placement Service Floor Plan Example; see also the PPS page at CareerPharm.com, where an interactive floor plan will be available beginning a month or two prior to MCM); however, certain areas will be restricted before the main event.

 Losing your badge can have irreparable consequences. Keep it in a safe place when you're not wearing it.

Once you decide which programs to pursue, keep an organized list of what each has to offer and why you chose it. Scheduling interviews will be less complicated if you are able to complete the task early. As PPS approaches, sites will have filled interview slots or may only have a few available times to choose from. Therefore, it would be good practice to e-mail the contact person for each program once you have determined the program has elements that appear to meet your goals. Be professional and complimentary of the program in your e-mail and request an interview time if available as discussed in Chapter 3: Contacting Residency and Fellowship Directors. Creation of a spreadsheet with your interview schedule to avoid double-booking is advisable. This can also keep you organized during PPS. When creating your schedule, attempt to allocate 30 minutes between each 30- to 60-minute interview to allow yourself time to reflect on your recent experience. This will allow you to write down key points (e.g., what you liked, what you did not), relax, grab some water, use the restroom, and find the next interview without running late. Additionally, interviewers may start late or end late, so you may not be in control of when the interview stops. This time cushion will also allow you to enjoy the rare occasion when you are in an immersive conversation with program representatives that extends beyond the scheduled time window without becoming nervous about your next appointment. If circumstances conspire and you do arrive late to an interview, simply apologize and then move on. Interviewers typically understand PPS is very busy and not everything always goes as planned. Of note, when making your schedule, consider interviewing with your top choice after you have interviewed with a few other programs. This can provide a chance to better understand the PPS processes before your big interview as well as help reduce any initial nerves.

> **Creating a spreadsheet of your Personnel Placement Service schedule either on paper or a digital device such as your smartphone or tablet pc will make life easier for you.** <

> **If you arrive late to a Personnel Placement Service interview, simply apologize and move on.** <

Take into consideration that PPS will overlap with other MCM events and may become your primary experience at the conference. Overlap with the Residency Showcase should not be ignored if you are interested in learning about programs that are not participating in PPS or that you only have access to through the Residency Showcase. If you are particularly interested in a program and have an interview scheduled through PPS, visiting the Residency Showcase of the institution in addition to your interview is appreciated and will accentuate your interest. Throughout your day(s) participating in PPS, you will most likely be asked similar questions for each interview and will be speaking for a prolonged period of time. Likewise, interviewers will be repeating information with multiple applicants. This can make for an exhausting experience for those on both sides. Take this into account by listening closely when interviewers speak and thank them for their time.

If you are particularly interested in a program and have an interview scheduled through Personnel Placement Service, visiting the Residency Showcase booth of that institution in addition to your interview is appreciated and will accentuate your interest.

An e-mail driven system is utilized to provide communication between employers and applicants. Computers are available on-site if you need to check messages while at the meeting; however, most of the communication will be completed prior to the meeting. Check the site at minimum twice daily to ensure you have not missed an important message. This should be preferably done at midday to allow some time in the afternoon to schedule any catch up meeting with a program of interest and in the evening to prepare for the following day, if needed. If you only check once in the evening, you risk the chance of missing an opportunity.

When you enter the PPS section, you will notice each institution is assigned a numbered booth (or booths). The size of the booth does not indicate the size of the program; however, large booths generally represent institutions recruiting for multiple positions. Booth numbers and names of the institution are posted on each booth and within the guide-book provided at the entrance to PPS. Interviews are generally conducted inside the booth, which contains a small table with a few chairs enclosed by a curtain. There are also a table and chairs directly outside of each booth, which may be utilized for the session.

During the interview, be sure to focus on the interviewer(s) and avoid becoming distracted by the bustling noise and what is happening around you. Shake hands and introduce yourself to each interviewer you meet. Feel free to ask if they have an area of specialty. This can provide a better understanding of what questions they may be able to answer (and what subjects to avoid). Never downplay a specialty because it is not something you are interested in. Each practitioner has specific passions and plays a vital role in the healthcare system. It is important to show respect and avoid negativity. Maintain a professional demeanor throughout the one-on-one interview. If your interviewer is relaxed, feel free to take queues from their behavior; however, always maintain your composure and keep up your guard. Answer questions with full sentences, being complete but concise in your answers. As your interview comes to a close, request the contact information for the person you have been speaking with as a route for asking more specific questions post-PPS.

> When greeting an interviewer, give a firm handshake with a two-time, upward-downward movement. More on this topic in Chapter 6: Interview Day.

Some programs may make last-minute changes and may not be able to obtain a booth or fit you into their interview schedule. This may lead to a program requesting to meet an applicant outside of the PPS time and area, such as at a coffee shop or food court. This is not uncommon and does not indicate you have been relegated to a less desirable interview slot. Such meetings, however, should be conducted in a professional location, and it is not common to be asked to meet employers at a location that is far from PPS, the MCM, or off-site.

Finally, you may not be remembered by everyone you meet in the Residency Showcase as there are a vast number of applicants present. However, you will be remembered if you interview at PPS. Do not feel you must leave a significant impression, but show that you are interested, intelligent, and qualified to add to the employer's department. With the right amount of preparation, professionalism, and positivity, PPS is guaranteed to be a productive experience.

AFTER THE SESSIONS

While You Are Still at the ASHP MCM

In addition to the Residency Showcase and PPS, there are other opportunities applicants may take advantage of during the MCM. Evening receptions may be offered by pharmacy programs or other institutions to provide networking opportunities to alumni, employees, and business partners. If you are invited to attend, do not be afraid to introduce yourself to other attendees and strike up a conversation about your current interests and future plans. This can be a great source for advice and insight, but beware the possibility of bias, as postgraduate training programs can change dramatically from year to year. Also, if your initial plans do not yield the desired result, this may serve as a resource to connect with other employment opportunities. At these events limit your consumption of alcoholic beverages and use sound judgment.

 Evening receptions and poster sessions are situations where business cards are handy to distribute.

Another opportunity during the MCM are the poster sessions. RPDs, preceptors, residents, fellows, and students all have an opportunity to present their work at various times throughout the MCM. Visiting a member from a program of interest as they present their poster can provide more face-time, which may be especially noteworthy if you missed them during the Residency Showcase or PPS. It is important to recognize and discuss their project; however, if they have the time (which presenters frequently do), it is also acceptable to discuss their specific institution and program at this venue. If you are presenting a poster during the meeting you definitely want to invite residency representatives to visit your work. This provides another opportunity to highlight your accomplishments and make an additional impression. Do not overlook the benefits of networking at the poster sessions; however, the scholarship presentations remain the primary focus of this time and should not be overshadowed by exploring residency opportunities.

Following the ASHP MCM

After returning home from the MCM, you should have a good idea of which programs you are most interested in. Reviewing the information collected during your visit and reconciling this with the qualities you are looking for in a program will help narrow your selections. At this point, it is important to both follow up with the programs you encountered during the MCM, as outlined in Chapter 3: Contacting Residency and Fellowship Directors and Chapter 7: Following Up After the Interview, but also to move forward with preparing your application materials. The time between the conclusion of the MCM (early December) and the beginning of application deadlines (late December) will pass quickly. Do not delay in finalizing your list of programs, becoming aware of application deadlines, and carefully completing each component of your application.

Summary

Attendance at the MCM includes multiple opportunities for those pursuing postgraduate training and allows applicants to gather vital information, network, and further explore and discover the many available options in one convenient location. Participation in the Residency Showcase or PPS provides direct access to those involved in providing residency training and conducting residency recruitment. Applicants who prepare in advance and take advantage of the various activities at the MCM are rewarded with additional knowledge about each program and the chance to leave a positive impression on those they encountered. Both will prove beneficial while entering the next phase of the residency application process. If you go, stay positive, perform your due diligence, make a plan, and stay focused.

 KEY LESSONS

- The ASHP Midyear Clinical Meeting encompasses many events, including the Residency Showcase and Personnel Placement Service.

- The Residency Showcase and Personnel Placement Service are designed to connect postgraduate training applicants with representatives from hundreds of programs in one venue.

- The Residency Showcase is primarily geared toward postgraduate year-1 and postgraduate year-2 pharmacy residency applicants.

- Personnel Placement Service is highly utilized by those seeking a postgraduate year-2 pharmacy residency, fellowship, and/or post-training employment.

- Preparation and organization are key elements to a successful experience and should not be taken lightly.

- Consider initially exploring a wide range of programs and do not limit yourself.

REFERENCES

1. Fotis M. Advice for residency applicants going to the Midyear Clinical Meeting. *Am J Health-Syst Pharm.* 2006;63(19):1787, 1791.

2. ASHP: The Midyear 2011 residency program online listing. Available at http://www.ashp.org/Midyear2011/ResidencyShowcase/Residency-Program-Listing.aspx. Accessed March 26, 2012.

3. Careerpharm online. Available at http://www.careerpharm.com/. Accessed March 26, 2012.

4. Mancuso C, Paloucek F. Understanding and preparing for pharmacy practice residency interviews. *Am J Health-Syst Pharm.* 2004;61(16):1686-1689.

FORMALLY APPLYING AND GETTING READY FOR A PHARMACY RESIDENCY INTERVIEW

Milap C. Nahata, PharmD, MS

Joshua Caballero, PharmD, BCPP

After arriving home from the ASHP Midyear Clinical Meeting (MCM) or when evaluating all the programs you are interested in applying to, an important question you may struggle with is, "How many programs should I formally submit applications to?" The answer is complicated and most professors will offer you venerable and ivory tower answers, such as, "As many as you feel necessary," "As many programs as you found that met your criteria," etc. Ideally, you want to formally apply to as many programs as possible that match your interests in order to increase your chances of securing interviews; however, there are also practical concerns to keep in mind. For example, consider the amount of time and money you will have to devote to traveling if you plan on applying in different cities and states. This willingness to move will likely increase your options for residencies tremendously, but will have to be accounted for in terms of your available resources to travel for the interviews.

 Saving money throughout pharmacy school—and having February off—will assist you in simplifying your interview schedule, thus allowing you to interview at many more places.

FORMALLY APPLYING TO PROGRAMS

From our unpublished data, approximately 66% of the sites you submit applications to will offer you an interview. However, the range of securing such interviews varies widely (0% to 100%). We have had students submit 15 applications and get no interviews and we have had students submit 12 applications and receive 11 interviews despite similar grades and level of

extracurricular activity. Given this, a good number to consider applying to is
10 to 15 programs. While the number may seem high, this means you may
receive seven to nine interviews. If you secure more interviews than you can
travel to, you can always send a polite and direct e-mail declining the
invitation to interview. Lastly, provided they have the essential qualities you
are looking for, consider applying to a wide variety of programs such as
programs affiliated with an academic teaching center, community hospital,
specialty hospital (e.g., pediatric hospital), and government-affiliated
institution. Having a target pool with a wide variety of programs allows you
more flexibility in selecting those you want to interview at and ultimately
will provide you a longer list for your match (see Chapter 8: Matching).

 **If you do not consider yourself a "top" applicant, you may
consider applying to more programs. However, even if you feel
you are the ideal applicant for a program, do not limit yourself to
only one to three programs.**

Submit Application Materials

When preparing your application materials, make sure you pay careful
attention to detail. Every year, there are subsets of applications that are not
considered because they are incomplete. Common reasons include that the
residency program director (RPD) did not receive the forms completely
filled out (including your signature), transcripts are missing, and letters of
recommendations are not received. While you may not be able to completely control if letters of recommendation are submitted on time, there are
some steps you can take to increase the likelihood. Approach professors
and employers in advance (e.g., early November) to let them know you will
be applying to residency positions; inform them that you will supply them
with a list as soon as you return from the MCM. Upon return from the
MCM, make a list of the programs you will be applying to and supply a
packet to your recommenders as soon as possible. The packet should
include your curriculum vitae (CV), personal statement (PS), and a list of
the programs you are applying to. In the event that the program is not
using Pharmacy Online Residency Centralized Application Service (PhOR-
CAS), be sure to include addresses or e-mails of where to send the letters.
Providing typed address labels that can easily be placed on the envelopes

for programs not in PhORCAS will eliminate the potential for error and make the recommenders' job much easier.

If a residency program is requesting three letters of recommendation, ask four recommenders to send letters to that specific program. In the event of an unforeseen variable (e.g., lost letter, family emergency, vacation), you should still be covered with three. If a program receives four letters, that's okay—better more than less in this case. You can always send a courtesy reminder e-mail to your recommenders that letters are due in case they have not informed you they have submitted or sent their letters. Also, some RPDs may e-mail you and state they have received two of three letters (and provide names of those who have submitted their letters). This will allow you to contact the recommender and make arrangements, if necessary (*hopefully, if you followed the advice above, this won't be the case*). The good news is that as mentioned in Chapter 1: Preparing to Compete for a Pharmacy Residency, ASHP will be introducing PhORCAS, which will allow applicants to streamline the above process and make life easier for everyone. However, please note that you may be applying to programs that are nonaccredited or did not register with the system. Therefore, make sure you know which programs are registered for to avoid any confusion when applying.

 Professors and employers should be approached regarding letters of recommendation during the beginning of November. Additionally, when asking people for letters of recommendations, make sure you ask for a *favorable* letter.

After formally submitting all your applications and delivering all materials to your recommenders, find a couple of days to relax and decompress. There may be a two- to six-week period between submitting all your applications and receiving invitations to interview. The anxiety regarding whether you will secure interviews can be daunting, but keep your emotions in check. If you have been following our advice and done your due diligence, your efforts should soon be rewarded.

YOU SECURED INTERVIEWS

Congratulations! You have secured interviews! Whether you have received
one or 10 interviews, it is important to be fully prepared. Now is the time
to think about how to prepare and determine the logistics of your visit(s).
Questions may include the following:

- What dates and for how long will I visit?
- How will I pay for the trip?
- What should I expect?
- What additional details should the program provide me?

As soon as you are invited to the interview, you should begin to
address all of these questions. The purpose of the following sections is to
offer vital recommendations to get you ready for a successful pharmacy
residency interview.

Find the Most Convenient Dates for Interviews

As you are granted interviews, show flexibility and consideration to
select the dates that are most convenient for the residency programs,
the preceptors with whom you are doing advanced pharmacy practice
experiences (APPEs), and finally for yourself. Before contacting the RPD
and your APPE preceptor to explore possible dates, it is best to have a
general idea of flight times and airfares or driving time. These logistical
details are important to address in advance to achieve efficiency in
scheduling various interviews. Similarly, this is another opportunity to
demonstrate to the program that you have desirable qualities of time
management, attention to detail, and organization. Failure to do your
due diligence on something as seemingly innocuous as making travel
plans may result in you scrambling to make last minute changes,
consequently inconveniencing the RPD, and ultimately making a
negative impression before you even arrive for the interview. Additionally, explore the possibility of doing multiple interviews during the
same trip. I have had some students who have coordinated a trip to a
city or state and interviewed at three sites in four days to save money

on airfare. Another option is not to schedule an APPE for February (as
mentioned in Chapter 1: Preparing to Compete for a Pharmacy Residency) to position yourself with maximum flexibility to accommodate most
requests.

**Send a courtesy e-mail to your advanced pharmacy practice
experience preceptor(s) reminding them of your potential
interviews for residencies during the month.**

**If possible, when making your schedule, consider interviewing
with your top choice(s) after you have interviewed with a few
other programs.**

Know the Program (and Its People)

This is among the most important factors to achieve success in an interview. You must know as much as possible about the strengths and limita-
tions of the residency program, and about the name and the track record of
the RPD as well as individuals participating in the interview process and
training residents at the site. Internet resources (e.g., institutional websites,
Google, PubMed) should be utilized to obtain information about the
hospital/clinic/university, residency program, and the achievements of the
RPD and preceptors. This will also allow you to see what specialty area
within their practice they focus on (e.g., diabetes in ambulatory care,
infectious disease in internal medicine). Review one to two of their latest
journal articles (preferably in their specialty area), so you gain some insight
about their contributions to the profession and the opportunities that may
exist for you. It is also useful to obtain information from the past and
current residents of the programs. You can obtain this information from
talking to them at the ASHP MCM, or the program may have a listing of
the current residents and their contact information on their website. Some

residency programs will even list their past residents, which you may be able to locate by performing another search. The goal of these key steps is to be well prepared and confident about why you are seeking this position and develop the most pertinent questions to ask during the interviews. Having no questions to ask will make you look unprepared or uninterested; therefore, consult the example questions in Appendix C: Potential Questions Asked During Residency Interviews, and Appendix F: Questions to Ask and Avoid When Interviewing, if you need help in developing your own.

Update and Review Your CV and Portfolio

Even though the CV and PS were shared earlier with the residency programs, it is important to update your CV with new information (e.g., work performed during latest APPE, special projects conducted, presentations made, papers accepted or published). More importantly, review your CV and PS so that you are ready to explain what was done and how those experiences make you a strong and unique applicant for their residency program. You should bring attention to and focus on the most impressive items (and what you are most proud of) when RPDs and interviewers are reviewing your CV and interviewing you. If you have created a portfolio, make sure to update and review it in preparation for your interviews in the event the RPDs and preceptors request to see it.

During an interview one of my former students focused on a specific drug monograph she had worked on. When discussing it, one of the interviewers was particularly interested in the topic. Having a hard copy of the monograph in her portfolio to share with the interviewer along with a detailed explanation (conveying understanding and enthusiasm) separated her from other interviewees. Please note that by sharing your portfolio you are opening yourself to being assessed on the portfolio; therefore, if using one, make sure it is aesthetically pleasing and that you have a firm understanding regarding the materials therein.

A portfolio is a professional binder that contains a hard or electronic copy of all your presentations, drug monographs, and posters to date. It is best to have two to three hard copies of each presentation in case one of the interviewers wants to keep a hard copy.

Prepare to Compose the Best Answers to the Expected and Tough Questions

There are endless books and articles covering different types of questions you may be asked in an interview. You should prepare to answer the standard and difficult interview questions described in Appendix C: Potential Questions Asked During Residency Interviews. Being honest and confident is just as important as being well prepared, as there may not be right or wrong answers to many questions or situations. How you respond to unexpected or difficult questions is the key.

Network and Practice Interviewing with Faculty or Preceptors

As a residency applicant, you should get to know at least some of your faculty and preceptors in the PharmD program to get additional tips and suggestions for good interview preparation. It is also good to practice interviewing with one or two preceptors so that some of the difficulties in answering questions can be overcome. At the very least, practicing with fellow classmates can also prepare you in the event you cannot schedule time with a preceptor. Some pharmacy programs are also offering seminars, or courses related to residency preparation.[1,2] Also, organizations such as ASHP, American Association of Colleges of Pharmacy (AACP), and American College of Clinical Pharmacy (ACCP) offer mock interviews at their regional and national meetings. Take advantage of those opportunities if you can. Or, if you are ambitious, develop and organize a mock interview session through an organization at your institution, if one does not exist.

Learn to project confidence and excellent interpersonal skills

Positive interpersonal skills and attitude are essential for teamwork and to achieve the goals of residency training. Thus, learn to project your confidence, not only in pharmacy knowledge and skills, but also in sharing your personal strengths as an individual. Your experiences in extracurricular and leadership activities should be highlighted during the interview process as opportunities arise. Be confident, but be careful not to come across as being "arrogant." Even though there are different perceptions of attitude among the various residency programs, there is a thin line to balance between what constitutes confidence and hubris. Constructive criticism regarding your mock interviews should help you in finding that balance. Additionally, having knowledge about the residency programs, RPDs, and the interviewers will help you establish a rapport with them at the time of interviews.

Get an Appropriate Dress or Suit, a Folder, and Carry a Positive Outlook

Dressing professionally is important in creating a positive impression of your judgment. It is a good practice to dress more conservatively with solid colors lacking excessive designs and flair. Perfume and jewelry should be minimal. This may help convey professionalism.

For men — wear a suit with a tie and dress shoes. Preferably, the suit should be blue, brown, or grey. Black is sometimes avoided; however, you can contrast it with a colorful (not garish) shirt/tie and look professional and fashionably chic. The tie should be professional (e.g., no cartoons, no political statements), and shoes should be polished.

For women — wear a business suit with a skirt or pants, or a conservative dress. Closed-toed shoes with a small heel, if needed (no stilettos) are recommended. Professional attire should not be low cut and panty hose should be worn when wearing a skirt (which should be knee level or below). Keep your makeup neutral and avoid bright colors. There is an exception to the color scheme rules. If you previously know that the RPD or preceptors dress with more color (from initial interaction during the MCM or APPEs), then you can take a chance if you feel you want to be different — especially to a site that is highly coveted and interviewing many competitive applicants. We like to call this a "high risk, high rewards" tactic.

> **You can have a tie or a scarf that is colorful and vibrant—as long as it doesn't draw too much attention.**

Metal facial jewelry including tongue rings should be removed. Even if you wear a nose ring for religious/cultural reasons, some programs may not understand. However, if a residency program does not have a favorable view on your nose ring, then this may not be the residency for you. Therefore, how you present yourself and how much conviction you have on wearing facial jewelry will be a personal decision (fashion vs. cultural). If you have tongue rings, take them out (yes we can see them and they can become distracting). Along with the metal motif comes the issue with wearing pharmacy pins, or what is commonly referred to as *flair.* You may wear up to two pins (some suggest no more than one). Preferable pins to wear include an academic society (e.g., Phi Lambda Sigma, Rho Chi) or a professional fraternity (e.g., Kappa Psi, Phi Delta Chi). Wearing an academic pin will subtly portray your leadership (Phi Lambda Sigma) or scholastic (Rho Chi) accomplishments whereas the fraternity pin may elicit icebreaking conversation ("Oh, you were a member of AZO. What was your favorite chapter activity?"). You should also be prepared to answer questions such as, "How involved were you with this organization?" or "Did you do or lead any special project with this group?"

A folder, briefcase, or attaché case with a few copies of your CV, portfolio (with two to three copies of key presentations or monographs), interview itinerary, directions, note pad, and pen should be prepared. Sleep well and consume no alcohol, onions, garlic, or strong curry the day before and on the day of the interview. You should also remember to think positively (*you would not be interviewing if they did not feel you were worthy*). Being relaxed and unstressed are important components of preparing well to maximize your performance in the interviews. Consider bringing nonpharmacy-related reading to keep your mind off the interview while you wait.

> **If you have a tablet computer (e.g., iPad), you are welcome to use it and take advantage of its functionality during interviews. However, be careful that you don't become enamored with it to the point of distraction.**

Overall, during the interview take notes, be proactive, ask appropriate questions, and avoid poor and unnecessary questions as described in Appendix F: Questions to Ask and Avoid When Interviewing. Asking thoughtful questions and taking notes are two clear signs of a prepared applicant. When applicants are given the chance, throughout or at the end of the interview, to pose questions and fail to do so, they are universally evaluated more poorly.

Prepare Your Presentation

Most interviews today require students to prepare and deliver a presentation. Sometimes programs will assign a specific topic, or format that they want you to follow. If this is not communicated by the program, it is appropriate to ask the RPD if there are specific requirements. However, when you are given the latitude, choose a topic you are genuinely enthusiastic about, have given a presentation on in the past (e.g., during a previous APPE), and feel confident discussing. Here are some tips for putting together your PowerPoint™ presentation:

- Choose a font size that will be clear, especially in the handouts. We usually recommend that students send the RPD a portable document format (PDF) file of their handouts instead of the PowerPoint™. This way, it has been perfectly formatted the way you want it and you do not have to worry if the formatting changes when someone converts and prints your handout.

- For the slide background choose neutral patterns and designs. Don't let it be overwhelming. Exception to the rule: you can use the "high risk, high rewards" approach as discussed with how to dress.

- Keep word count to a minimum. If you add too many words, the slides will look busy and it will appear as if you are *reading* your presentation. You will fall into that professor category you disliked, who read their slides during class as you sat there thinking, "Why am I sitting here when I can read." Instead, limit the word count and then as you present, you will be talking more than *reading*. You should also have notes on your presentations based on questions they may ask. You may write mechanism of actions, guidelines, monitoring parameters, and specific details you feel someone may ask you. Even though you may know, sometimes when asked during a presentation, you can get nervous and have a memory lapse. In this case, you can refer to your notes and answer appropriately.

■ Check spelling and punctuation. Spell check and double check that drug names and dosage regimens are correctly mentioned. Having these misspelled shows lack of attention to detail.

■ References should be pristine and consistent. Let us repeat—make sure your references are *perfect!* This means you have referenced correctly all of the presented data including any images you used from the Internet. We recommend the style of uniform requirements utilized by most peer-reviewed journals including *American Journal of Health-System Pharmacy, Annals of Pharmacotherapy,* and *Pharmacotherapy.* Having one reference with issues and the other missing the issue, or having the journal completely detailed in one reference but abbreviated in another again shows lack of attention to detail. If you use another style, be consistent! Also, remember to use primary literature for your information, not lay websites. Nothing kills a presentation more than getting to the references and seeing Wikipedia or blog pages. Additionally, try not to reference the DiPiro or Koda-Kimble textbooks. Instead, perform a literature search to find your own original studies. This again will show you took the extra step.

 For a one-stop shop of how to cite almost any biomedical resource, consider the free online book by the National Library of Medicine, Citing Medicine (http://www.ncbi.nlm.nih.gov/books/ NBK7256/).

■ Practice, practice, practice! Ideally, record yourself presenting so that you can identify any distracting nuances such as saying "um," making odd gestures with your hands, rocking back and forth, and the speed at which you talk. It is humbling to watch oneself presenting. Practice alone or with classmates. Ask for honest and constructive feedback. Make sure to review and practice again a day before the presentation.

- Include pictures or diagrams that highlight the presentation and make it more appealing. Too much material and busy tables or figures that do not show or print well should be avoided. You could include them as a page-size appendix to the end of your presentation packet. That way when you are presenting, you can state, "If you look at the end of your handout, here is the diagram." This shows you took the time to make sure the entire presentation was readable and clear—you took the extra step.

- Make sure your presentation answers the "So what?" factor. Your presentation should have a clear meaning and takeaway for those attending your presentation. If, instead of 20–60 minutes to present, you only had *one* minute — what would you say?

> **Be smart when using pictures and images from the Internet. Make sure you use images that are not copyrighted. Some may allow you to use them if it is for educational purposes; however, make sure you reference the images.**

> **Convert your handouts (e.g., PowerPoint™, Word™) to portable document format (PDF) files. This way, it has been perfectly formatted by you.**

> **Make sure you have extra slides (either at the end or using the Hide Slide function) regarding a topic if you think someone may ask a more in-depth question than what your presentation time allotted you to present. This way, if the question is asked, you can use that slide to provide your answer.**

Practice for On-Site Patient Cases and Literature Evaluations

Some interviews may provide you with a patient case and give you anywhere from as little as five to as many as 60 minutes to dissect and present the case. Another exercise may be to receive a journal article and have 20 to 60 minutes to prepare an abstract for it or present a critique of it. In order to prepare for these scenarios, make sure to review common disease states and pharmacotherapy. Common disease states in ambulatory settings may include diabetes, hypertension, hyperlipidemia, depression, and thyroid disorders. Common disease states in inpatient settings include infectious diseases (e.g., pneumonia) or electrolyte disturbances (e.g., hypernatremia, hypokalemia). If you are applying at a specialty hospital (i.e., pediatrics) or a postgraduate year-2, ensure you review common conditions for that specific patient population. Make sure you review guidelines, monitoring parameters, target endpoints, and primary counseling points. When evaluating cases with multiple disease states, you should be able to rank the disease states that require immediate attention (e.g., heart attack versus hyperlipidemia). You may also wish to practice and time yourself for some of these exercises. Acquiring a case book (e.g., DiPiro's *Pharmacotherapy Casebook*) may be a great idea, not only to help you prepare for this section of the interview, but also to start preparing for the licensing examination as well. To prepare for a journal article evaluation, start with your notes from your literature evaluation or evidence-based medicine coursework and brush up on the statistical and methodological portions. You should be familiar with some of the more common tests (e.g., Chi square, t-test, analysis of variance [ANOVA]) and when each are appropriate to use. It is recommended that you practice by reading a few articles from reputable journals and then critique/evaluate them. This may be better done by forming groups of three to four students who are also pursuing a residency. The group can then select an article and take 30 minutes to read and prepare. Afterward, each of you can state your views on the article and see how each of you evaluated the study. There may be some other unexpected situations that arise during your interview. However, if you are well prepared, you will stay relaxed and confident in any situation.

Focus on What You Can Control

Despite securing interviews, you may start focusing on the negative—do not! It is critical not to waste any energy stressing about the programs that did not grant you an interview. This is unproductive and will cause you to waste time (at best) and damage your self-confidence (at worst). Scenarios along these lines that we have observed students struggling with include the following:

- Spending a third of their APPEs at a specific institution and feeling assured of an interview based on the feedback during their time there, but not being granted an interview.

- Questioning their own merit for even being able to complete a residency because they did not get an interview with a first-choice program they felt they connected with.

- Feeling ambushed because they secured multiple letters of recommendation from pharmacists at a specific institution, but then did not get an interview from that site or an explanation as to why.

There are a multitude of reasons why you may not have received an interview with a specific program and now is not the time to dwell on it or let it negatively impact your self-confidence. Again, you have to get over it and move on! Instead, draw your focus and attention to the programs that *did* grant you an interview. You did not come this far to focus on things you cannot control; again, focus on what you can control—how you perform the days of your interviews. Remember, out of the countless applications they reviewed, they found something in *your* application or in personally meeting you during the MCM that intrigued them enough to want to interview you. This is your time to shine!

 KEY LESSONS

- When asking professors or employers for letters of recommendation, make sure you ask well ahead of time, ask for a favorable letter, and provide all materials to them in a timely and organized fashion.

- Maintain as much flexibility as possible in your schedule to accommodate interviews.

- Wear a suit and avoid anything that will be too distracting. Remember, color is okay as long as it works to accentuate your suit and is not distracting.

- Practice interview questions with classmates, preceptors, or professors to help you get comfortable with the process.

- Practice other aspects of the interview process such as presentations, case dissections, or journal evaluations with classmates.

- Prepare questions for those who you are interviewing with.

- Do not dwell on that which you cannot control.

REFERENCES

1. Caballero J, Benavides S, Steinberg JG, et al. Development of a residency interviewing preparatory seminar. *Am J Health-Syst Pharm*. 2012;69(5):400-404.

2. Koenigsfeld CF, Wall GC, Miesner AR, et al. A faculty-led mock residency interview exercise for fourth-year doctor of pharmacy students. *J Pharm Pract*. 2012;25(1):101-107.

CHAPTER 6

INTERVIEW DAY

Andrew C. Seger, PharmD

Mary Amato, PharmD, MPH, BCPS

Many people are nervous on their interview day. It is a familiar response to new situations, especially when the stakes are high and the outcomes are uncertain. By preparing well in advance and thoughtfully examining what you wish to achieve, from a personal, professional, and societal perspective, your ultimate goals should be within your grasp. You should also understand that in the interview there are things that are out of your control, but your ability to be passionate, knowledgeable, and tactful during the interview process is always important to establishing a connection with the interviewer.

WHAT TO EXPECT/PREPARATION

All the previous chapters have prepared you for this day: The interview day! The interview is one of the last steps in the process of securing a residency or fellowship. The purpose of the interview is to primarily see if

- you can do the job;
- you get along with the group; and
- you will enjoy what you do.

The first bullet was partially answered with your curriculum vitae (CV) and personal statement (PS) and will be further elucidated during your presentation, patient case, exam, journal evaluation, or any other scholarly activity that may be presented. The second and third bullets allude to Robert Suttons' book, *The No Asshole Rule: Building a Civilized Workplace and Surviving One That Isn't.*[1] Generally most colleagues do not

Acknowledgment: The authors would like to thank Sarah P. Slight, MPharm, PhD, for her assistance in reviewing this material.

want to work with people who are not polite, cause complications or
turmoil, or make for a hostile work environment. Therefore, the interview
is extremely important to all involved and should be taken seriously. In our
opinion, the process of preparing for the interview should start at least six
months prior to the interview. It would be beneficial to start earlier by
gaining an understanding of what is in the market place (e.g., reviewing
residency programs that you are considering applying to in the middle of
your third professional year). You need to be clear with what your goals are
and make sure the site(s) you have applied to meet your criteria. In addition, networking with current residents or fellows, other pharmacy students, or through social networking sites such as LinkedIn® or ASHP
Connect (http://connect.ashp.org), can be a useful way of gaining an
effective insight into whether a site meets your educational goals and
whether it would be a good fit for you. In addition to learning about a site,
it is important to reflect on and prepare for potential questions about
yourself that you may be asked on interview day. If possible, as mentioned
earlier, you should also conduct practice interviews with other students,
preceptor, or faculty and obtain feedback to improve your interview skills.

While maintaining a clean social network, it is a great idea to use
a professional network such as LinkedIn®. Since pharmacy is a
small world, you just may get a foot in the door simply by
knowing someone.

Screening Interview

A screening interview may be required as an initial portion of the overall
interview process. These are usually done via telephone and sometimes
utilizing videoconferencing software such as Skype™. The phone interview
is more common and there may be more than one interviewer asking
questions. In both of these situations, you should make a list of your
educational goals and where you see yourself focusing your practice (i.e.,
internal medicine, infectious disease). You should also have some talking
points that are not covered in your CV or PS that will help the interviewer
better understand who you are as a person. Some examples of this might

be that you spent a summer in Cambodia working with patients infected with HIV; you might have spent 12 weeks in Boston working with an integrated delivery network to update clinical knowledge in their information system related to drug–drug interactions. Those community service projects or advanced pharmacy practice experiences (APPEs) that have shaped and inspired your development should be communicated to help the interviewer(s) understand if you are a good fit for their site.

INTERVIEW DAY

It is important to arrive on time to your interview, even if the interviewer is behind on their scheduled interviews. You may use this extra time to reflect on the different qualities and skills that you have to offer. The location of the interview can vary; some can take place at the site, while others may take place at a conference where many external distractions often exist. Performing a dry run of the interview will allow you to be more confident, better prepared to accommodate potential distractions, and more at ease. In addition, you are more likely to have a smooth interview process and be able to more effectively communicate your achievements and experiences to the interviewer.

 Practice interviewing with other students, preceptors, or faculty. Give and accept feedback.

BEHAVIOR

How you behave in the interview is of critical importance; it is typically used as a means to gauge how you will interact with members of the team at the site of the training program. It is vital for you to remain composed at all times. While you hope to be both polite and passionate in describing who you are and what your goals are, the feedback you received when practicing interviews should have allowed you to modify your behavior to more finely attain that balance. Avoid negative remarks about your previous experiences, avoid criticizing individuals or geographical areas, and try to remain positive and optimistic when communicating your goals. Good training sites seek to create a culture of positivity and may eliminate applicants who would jeopardize that goal. Another way of looking at a less than satisfactory experience is to understand what you learned about yourself and others and how you would seek to create new positive outcomes from a previously negative experience. In terms of behavior, you might state this in the interview as, "I learned something new from a less than ideal experience..." Remember, *how you frame your experiences can reveal just as much about you as the experiences you are conveying*.

Appropriateness of Behaviors

Greeting

The greeting is the launching pad for your interview and you should smile, make eye contact when introducing yourself, and shake hands firmly. Nothing kills an interview more than a "dead fish" hand shake. If you are not familiar with a "dead fish" handshake, it's because you are probably using one. A useful tip to help reduce sweating palms is to use an alcohol-based hand rub. One or two shakes of the hand are sufficient to greet. When meeting multiple persons in an interview (e.g., during a group interview) ensure that you make every effort to shake each person's hand during the introductions. In the past, one of us had a female applicant that shook the hands of only the males in the group interview room. Whether it was intentional or not, that omission in protocol created discontent and despite performing well during her interview she did not receive a high ranking. While understanding that different cultures have differing levels of greeting protocol, this is a professional interaction in the United States, designed for mutual benefit to both parties.

Eye Contact

The use of eye contact is important in many aspects of human interactions, including as a marker for effective communication with patients.[2] It is an important skill while giving oral presentations and perhaps more important in the interview process. The use of eye contact is most appropriate when you are trying to instill an important point during the interview. However, there is no need to add more dramatic effects (e.g., opening your eyes wider than normal to establish eye contact). This is likely to have a negative impact on the interviewer(s) and should be avoided.

THE INTERVIEW

Applicant interviews are often set up with only one interviewer, but the possibility of having multiple interviewers on a panel is not unusual. There are different nuances between the two formats such as flow between the participants but the goal remains the same for all parties involved. The desired outcome for you is to better understand if your goals are in line with that of the site, to better understand the culture of the site, and to think about how the two previous goals combine to provide postgraduate education to reach your career goals. The goals for us as interviewers are similar, but we also assess if you fit the overall structure of the training program. If you are invited for an on-site interview you will want to ask about what a usual or typical interview at the site would entail, who you might meet with, and what you might be asked to do, such as an oral presentation (see Chapter 5: Formally Applying and Getting Ready for a Pharmacy Residency Interview).

Behavior During a One-on-One Interview

The one-on-one interview is easiest from a focus point of view. Some of the points you need to communicate:

- Why do you want to come here?
- What can you do for us?
- Will you fit in?
- What makes you different from other applicants?

Conveying the answers to these issues in a concise way will benefit you. Every person is likely to answer these questions differently. It is essential that you articulate clearly what you will bring to the site and that you wish to be a part of their success. Since you are delivering the message to a single person, make sure that your eyes don't wander too far from the face of the interviewer. Remember to be prepared to ask the interviewer questions about the program. By asking questions that are thoughtful and engaging, you will demonstrate your critical thinking skills.

Asking Questions

Toward the end of the interview, you may be asked if you have any further questions. This question can always be used to your advantage. However, do not ask questions that could be easily answered from the site's webpage. At best, it illustrates a lack of awareness of a basic resource about the program you are espousing strong interest in; at worst, it's an indicator of lack of preparation for the interview. Instead take this opportunity to pose questions that demonstrate a characteristic you wish to highlight (e.g., attention to detail) and reveal an insightful approach to the nature of your queries. An example of a question may be, "I have taken the GRE and am thinking about getting my Master's in Public Health. What resources do you have available to potentially assist me in this?" Taking notes during pre-interview tours and during the process can help you formulate site-specific questions. If you are unable to do this or do not get the opportunity to do so, you can always fall back on a core set of general residency questions. If the tone of the interview becomes more personable (e.g., you are asked what you do for fun), a possible question might be, "I have heard and read many things about the River Walk and Diez y Seis de Septiembre festival in San Antonio, but can you tell me more about the city?" Other thoughtful questions may include, "What is your affiliation with The University of Texas at San Antonio's Institute for Health Disparities Research?" or "I have read that there are some innovative programs to increase access to preventive care. Can you tell me about how your medical center is involved?"

Behavior During Group Interviews

Group interviews are a team approach to evaluating applicants. During the interview you must remain cognizant of all of the interview participants, although some of the interviewers may seem less engaged in the interview process. It is advantageous to direct some of your responses to other members of the group, in addition to the questioner, as a way of engaging other individuals. This also allows you to potentially connect to that person even though they are less interactive in the interview process. The audience in the group interview may be smaller than typical for a clinical oral presentation, but the same presentation skills there should be used here. An example is that you need to "work the room" and not only focus on a single individual, such as the residency program director. This process will also help demonstrate your confidence in speaking to others, indicating your potential for using your communication skills to persuade health care colleagues about important patient care and clinical issues.

Asking Questions During Group Interviews

The process is similar as described for the one-on-one interview; however, as the number of persons in the group interview might be three or even more you may need to write down the questions so that you would have at a minimum one question for each interviewer. If you do a number of dry runs, you may have the ability to remember all of the questions you feel you need to ask, but by writing them down, you might be able to generate new questions during the interview. Some applicants' style may require reflection time to effectively answer questions during the interview, so it is key that the dry-run process is also used to potentially limit dead air time during the interview. The best way to approach this issue therefore is an individualized process. By practicing beforehand, you will have a smoother presentation and be more comfortable.

CONSIDERATIONS FOR ALL INTERVIEWS

Conduct During the Interview

The applicant should look at the overall interview process as an alternate way of learning. It is not didactic, such as a lecture; it is not learning similar to a clinical APPE, but learning about oneself and others in the professional world. As part of this process, you also grow in terms of your knowledge and skill at interviewing. Consideration and empathy in the healthcare that you provide for patients is essential to your professional practice, but it is also of great importance as part of the interview process. Although the ultimate goal of the interview is to receive an offer from the residency or fellowship program (or in the case of postgraduate year-1 to match), it is helpful to reflect on your overall experience during your interview for possible future applications.

You should take notes, but not copious notes, during your interview and after the interview has ended you should debrief either by yourself or with someone else. This allows you to record immediate impressions for later. If you have many interviews close to one another, it may be difficult to do this debriefing and you may forget details that are important to you.

Answering Questions

You should be prepared to answer questions (see Appendix C: Potential Questions Asked During Residency Interviews). These are sometimes difficult questions to answer, but by being prepared you will be able to inform the interviewer of who you are and your overall outlook in terms of your career. If during the interview you are informed that there has been a change in location, a change in the focus of the residency that does not match your interest, you should continue to be polite and answer all questions that are asked of you. After the interview, it is helpful to reflect again on whether the site is the best fit for you. In addition, follow-up e-mails are appropriate even though you may not see the site as a good landing spot for you (see Chapter 3: Contacting Residency and Fellowship Directors).

Difficult questions or difficult interviewers need to be dealt with as professionally as possible. You should continue with the interview, maintaining your composure. There are many types of interviewing styles and some of them might not match your philosophy, but you should proceed professionally. If you feel that the interviewer(s) have treated you in an unprofessional manner, then the site is most likely not for you.

Summary

There are many factors affecting potential career pathways in pharmacy. The opening of many new schools of pharmacy (thus an increased number of graduating pharmacists in the marketplace) and a sluggish world economy over the last four years have contributed to a much tighter market for both pharmacy jobs and postgraduate pharmacy training. While the number of residency positions has grown, the number of applicants is growing faster than the number of new positions. There are also new opportunities in research, informatics, and in accountable care organizations such as medical homes, where pharmacy practice is very tightly focused on a team approach of providing healthcare to patients, ultimately increasing effectiveness and safety of care, while reducing overall costs.

The interview process is a place where you as an applicant can differentiate yourself from others applying for these limited positions. Preparation is key and will give you the best chance of reaching your career and educational goals. Although positions in traditional pharmacy practice settings are more limited, there are also new opportunities in research. This will allow you the ability to provide essential healthcare services to patients while working with the healthcare team. Good luck!

 KEY LESSONS

- To be successful at interviewing, be sure to enlist friends, significant others, and possibly faculty members to help you practice and obtain useful feedback.

- Remain positive, enthusiastic, and composed at all times as the interviewer is gauging how you will fit into their specific setting.

- Phone interviews demand the same behavior and seriousness as an on-site interview.

- Regardless of your cultural background, be sure to greet all interviewers with a firm handshake and appropriate eye contact.

- Remember, you are interviewing the residency/fellowship as well, so be sure to get all of your questions regarding the program answered.

REFERENCES

1. Sutton RI. *The No Asshole Rule: Building a Civilized Workplace and Surviving One That Isn't.* New York, NY: Hachette Book Group; 2007.

2. Gorawara-Bhat R, Cook MA. Eye contact in patient-centered communication. *Patient Educ Couns.* 2011;82(3):442-447.

CHAPTER 7

Following Up After the Interview

Jose A. Rey, PharmD, MS, BCPP

You have just finished the interview with the residency or fellowship program and are now wondering, "What's next?" As soon as possible—perhaps at the airport or on the airplane—while the information, details, and names are fresh in your memory, start writing and sending thank-you e-mails. Why send thank-you notes? It is considered standard professional etiquette to send a thank-you note by e-mail to the principal interviewers almost immediately after the interview. These decision makers usually include the residency program director (RPD), preceptors of core rotations, director of the pharmacy department, department chair or dean if the site is at a pharmacy program, and even the current resident(s) of the program if they were involved in the interview process. Your e-mail should be brief, thanking the interviewer for their time, and could also include a detail pertaining to the time spent with that person and any clarification that you feel may be needed. It usually indicates your continued interest in their program; however, even if you're not interested in the program after the interview, the pharmacy world is surprisingly small and you should be aware that *you are always interacting with a network*. Both politeness and rudeness will be remembered. Also be aware that people at a program do talk to each other, so make every effort not to copy and paste the same thank-you to everyone there. The same dangers exist for changing just the name on a thank-you e-mail as with the contact e-mails discussed in Chapter 3: Contacting Residency and Fellowship Directors.

Pros and Cons of the Handwritten Note

The next step to consider is the handwritten note. Completion of this aspect of post-interview protocol is no longer universally recommended as it has somewhat been replaced by the thank-you notes delivered via e-mail. However, there are definitely still RPDs who consider the handwritten note as a fundamental indicator of a quality applicant who "takes that extra step." Alternately, other RPDs view receipt of a handwritten note that echoes a previously sent e-mail as a redundant time waster for them during the busiest part of the year. Unfortunately, there is no way to be certain if the RPD is a traditionalist who considers the handwritten note a necessity or the non-traditionalist RPD who considers your duty satisfactorily discharged after the e-mail. While there is no definitive answer, it is worth mentioning that a traditionalist who does not receive a handwritten note is apt to take far more notice than a non-traditionalist who is mildly annoyed by having received the same thank-you twice. Ultimately, you may have to make some situation-dependent decisions here as you will throughout the process of trying to secure a residency or fellowship.

 It is *always* important to send a thank-you e-mail. However, the necessity of a handwritten thank-you note is debatable.

If you do choose to send a handwritten note, keep in mind that for a traditionalist RPD, the handwritten note symbolizes your extra effort, thoughtfulness, and attention to detail. Alternately, it presents them with another opportunity to evaluate your candidacy. So make sure you are capitalizing on this opportunity to impress, not undercutting your positive interview by failing to observe convention and/or demonstrating poor judgment with the handwritten note. Before writing the note, you will need to acquire stationery (or heavier quality paper) and make sure you allot adequate time to carefully craft it—especially if the legibility of your handwriting has degenerated during pharmacy school. Also, bigger and more are not always better. The note does not have to be on full-size letter head; the small ones can be just as effective. In fact, your note should be both brief and simple (e.g., no fancy Hallmark cards). Otherwise, the same guidance for content and composition for e-mails applies to the handwritten note. Regardless of what type of culture of gift-giving that you come from, please remember that neither this note nor any other communication should contain a gift. Your well-intentioned token of appreciation may instead be interpreted as unprofessional, or in the case of federal institutions, possibly unethical.

Do not send gifts to program directors or anyone you have interviewed with.

 If sending a handwritten note, avoid inappropriate postage and address stickers. Remember to keep a sense of professionalism in all aspects.

FOLLOW-UP ACTIVITIES

If further information was requested (e.g., copy of the poster that you recently presented, an article that you published) or perhaps a part of your application packet was misplaced or not received, then, as soon as possible, attend to those requests by the fastest route available. This process should, ideally, go both ways. Remember that you are interviewing the program as much as they are interviewing you. You may have had a question for which the answer was not readily available (e.g., availability of a particular rotation/training experience). These questions are perfectly acceptable for you to follow-up with a phone call or e-mail so as to resolve the question and better inform your decision on whether to rank the program or not (see Chapter 8: Matching).

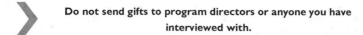 **Do not try to fake an answer during the interview. If you do not know, say so. You can always follow-up with an e-mail.**

Research any questions you could not answer on the spot, and send a specific answer to the questioner at the earliest available time. Please do not cut and paste the information, use Wikipedia, or use a blog as your source to answer the question. Use established and referenced guidelines or primary literature to support your answer, and remember to *use your own words*. Using e-mail is fine for this kind of follow-up activity. This action alone may be the difference that tips the decision in your favor, or at least speaks to your effort, willingness to resolve a question, and follow-up skills that will separate you from the pack of other applicants.

During one residency cycle, I had two applicants that were very close on paper (e.g., grade point average, curriculum vitae, extra-curricular activities) along with their general performance and impressions during the interview. During the interview a preceptor (who was not the RPD) had asked both applicants various questions, including esoteric ones, or those more difficult to answer. Soon after interviewing both of them, the RPD reported ambivalence between the two applicants, thinking both had performed in a similar fashion. However, one of the applicants, who did not know the answer to a question regarding a drug interaction during the interview, sent a detailed, correct answer to the interviewer soon afterward. This single action is what tipped the scales in favor of that applicant. Again, interviewers do not expect you to know the answer to every single question, but if you cannot answer a question, follow-up!

 Sometimes difficult questions are asked to observe the applicant under pressure, test the depth of their knowledge, and see if they can admit to not knowing an answer and what to do in that specific situation.

How and When to Inquire Regarding Your Applicant Status

After the interview, you typically start thinking about how well you performed: "Did I represent myself the way I wanted to?"..."Did they like me?"..."Do I like them?"..."Should I call?"..."Did they say 'Don't call us, we'll call you' or give me any timeline for a follow-up or status check such as, 'If you don't hear from us in one week, then give us a call or send us an e-mail'?" Many programs may thank you for your time after the interview and not have any further contact with you, leaving you with the question of how to rank the program or how to proceed if you are not in the Match program (e.g., nonaccredited residencies, fellowships, Scramble inter-views). The program may give you a specific date or a general statement like, "Expect a call from us next week."

For programs that are participating in the Match, it is not appropriate to ask the RPD or anyone affiliated with the residency how you fared and whether or not they will rank you (see Chapter 8: Matching). However for nonaccredited programs and fellowships, different rules apply. First, follow instructions. Hopefully, they gave you a guideline, or you remembered to ask about it at the end of your interview. If you interviewed on a Friday, then "next week" doesn't necessarily mean they will call you on Monday even if it is technically within the next week. Restrain yourself and wait until next Friday (or even the following Monday) before you make that phone call or send an e-mail regarding the status of your application and ask if they need anything else from you. The program will usually provide this type of information; however, a program with a large number of applicants may not contact you again after the interview. If not instructed about a follow-up from the program, you should inquire regarding their practice or expectations. Ideally, you found out what to expect from the program and what they expect from you post-interview. However, remember that the thank-you letter (e-mail and/or handwritten note) is the exception to any rules. They will not mention it, but send it anyway.

 Questions about a program's follow-up practice or expectations might be good ones for current residents, since they went through the process most recently.

THE (RARE) SECOND INTERVIEW OR MEETING

On the rare occasion that the first interview enabled you to separate from the group, but did not lead to a final decision, a second round of discussions may help to narrow the field or make the final decision. This second round is likely to occur via phone or videoconference—especially if the applicants are not local. As previously mentioned, be as accommodating as possible even if asked for a lunch meeting or conference call. Your ability to accommodate their schedule and address their needs or concerns will be noted by the program and may push you up the rankings. As mentioned in Chapter 6: Interview Day, be sure you know everyone in the room, at the table, or on the other end of that conference call (write down names on a notepad). Be sure to conduct yourself professionally, as you did in the first interview. Also, be careful about being or acting too familiar with the interviewer(s) during this second round of discussions and follow-up. Personalizing the interview may cause you to reduce your professional tone and address the interviewer(s) by their first name. You may also feel able to make a joke believing a different level of relationship now exists between yourself and the program's representatives, especially if significant time was spent with someone during the first interview and a level of comfort and relaxed attitude was created. Being relaxed and comfortable speaking to the interview group is good whether it is in the first or second interview; however, avoid overt familiarity and possible inappropriate comments that may come out because of it.

 KEY LESSONS

- Send a thank-you e-mail.
- Be aware of the situation-dependent decisions you must make during the process, such as sending a handwritten thank-you note.
- Address any questions raised during the interview and use your own words when formulating your response.
- Correct any mistakes you realize were made or said.
- Maintain a professional demeanor at all times.
- Inquire about the program's procedures for follow-up contact after the interview.

CHAPTER 8

MATCHING

Shara Elrod, PharmD, BCACP
Deanne L. Hall, PharmD, BCACP

Now that you have completed your on-site residency or fellowship interviews, sent thank-you letters (via e-mail and/or a handwritten note), and
submitted any supplemental materials, it is time to decide where you feel
you will fit the best, shine the most, and achieve your predetermined goals
and expectations. This chapter will help guide you through the residency
Match process so you can compile your program rank order list to secure
the best possible fit for residency training. Take out all of your interview
notes and get started!

NAVIGATING THE RESIDENCY MATCHING PROGRAM

The ASHP Residency Matching Program (RMP), otherwise known as the
Match, is managed by National Matching Service (NMS) Inc., and designed
to link residency applicants with ASHP-accredited postgraduate year-1
(PGY-1) and postgraduate year-2 (PGY-2) residency programs (http://
www.natmatch.com/ashprmp/).[1] The purposes of the RMP are twofold
with the first being to provide applicants and programs with the best
opportunity to seek out their true preferences, rather than making decisions under pressure (e.g., multiple offers with limited time) or with
incomplete information (e.g., an institution making hiring decisions
without a complete pool of applicants). Secondly, the RMP is designed to
ensure that applicants accept offers extended by programs.

Eligibility—Programs

You will have likely already made the decision on whether or not to apply
to ASHP non-accredited programs, but only programs that are ASHP-
accredited or in the process of becoming accredited (precandidate status)

are able to participate in the Match. This chapter will focus only on the process of the Match for accredited programs. If the residency you will be applying to is not currently accredited or applying for accreditation, it is best to ask the residency program director (RPD) early on for details regarding their particular program's application and selection process. Some nonaccredited programs will let you know of their decision prior to the Match to allow you to decide if you will still pursue programs in the Match. Be sure to ask RPDs when they will make their decisions, because they often have an accelerated timeline for interviewing and offering a position. If you accept a position prior to the Match, it is expected that you send a courtesy e-mail withdrawing your candidacy to the other programs you interviewed. The e-mail should be short and to the point: thank them for their time and consideration, that you have accepted a position, and to withdraw your application. This will go a long way since you may apply to their program again for a PGY-2 or pharmacy position after completing your PGY-1 residency. You may also cross paths again at meetings and possibly serve together on committees, and they will remember your actions, or lack thereof.

Eligibility—Applicants

To be eligible for the Match, you must have graduated or be in the process of graduating from an Accreditation Council for Pharmacy Education (ACPE)-accredited pharmacy program or be eligible for licensure. Foreign graduates must present a copy of their Foreign Pharmacy Graduate Examination Committee (FPGEC) certificate or a copy of each of their pharmacy licenses to be eligible for the Match. Applicants who are interested in a PGY-2 training program must either have completed a PGY-1 training program or be in the process of completing PGY-1 training. Applicants who are interested in a PGY-2 program, but who have not completed PGY-1 training may apply for exemption by submitting a curriculum vitae (CV) to ASHP provided they are licensed in the United States and have practiced for at least three years. For both PGY-1 and PGY-2 programs participating in the Match, you must apply, independently of the RMP, to each individual residency program to be considered for a position.

Deadlines and Registration

Early on during your information gathering process, it is a good idea to become familiar with dates and deadlines relating to the Match. Important deadlines include Match registration opening and closing dates, rank orders and withdrawals, submission opening and closing dates, and release of Match results. The dates and deadlines are available and continually updated on the ASHP RMP website (http://www.natmatch.com/ashprmp/).[1]

Applicant Agreement

As a part of registering for the Match, you are signing an applicant agreement, which outlines the rules for applicants agreeing to participate in the RMP. It is important to take time prior to registering for the Match to review these rules carefully, as this applicant agreement is binding. Any violation of the applicant agreement can be reported by either the NMS or by programs themselves to ASHP, which can impose penalties on applicants such as precluding applicants from pursuing ASHP-accredited residencies at any point in the future. One of the most important pieces of the agreement states that you must report to any program to which you are matched, even if it is not your preferred program. This stipulation makes it all the more important for you to rank only those programs that you can actually see yourself integrating into and completing. If you are matched and believe you will not be able to report on the agreed upon day, even if it is due to circumstances beyond your control (e.g., family emergency), you should contact the RPD as soon as possible after the release of the Match results to discuss any possible arrangements that can be made.

Residency Matching Program Violations

It is also a violation of the applicant agreement to discuss how you will rank programs or ask the RPD how they plan to rank you. It is okay and encouraged to be enthusiastic (within reason) especially when it is the residency that you want as your number one; however, use sound judgment. In a traditional interviewing process it is customary for the applicant "to seal an interview" with a commitment from the interviewer as to the level of interest and next steps in the hiring process (actually, an interviewer will look for and expect this). However, this is a structured matching program and the rules are different. You may express your enthusiasm, but refrain from stating how you will rank them and avoid putting pressure on the RPD to commit. This pressure will not be viewed as a positive and may come across as pushy. On the flip side, do not be surprised if an RPD calls you near the end date for listing residency/applicant preferences to gauge your interest in their program and circumvent the system. This is technically a violation from the program. If this occurs, again use sound judgment. You may express enthusiasm and support (e.g., "Yes, I really enjoyed your program and came away impressed with how successful your past residents have been"), but refrain from giving a number (e.g., "Yes, you're my number one").

> **Do not discuss your rankings with anyone from a program.**

Ranking Residency Programs

After completing all your interviews, the rank order will be your most important decision. You must ask yourself not only what order to rank the programs to which you applied, but also if you want to rank the program at all. You may be tempted to rank a program for fear of not matching elsewhere, but you are under no obligation to rank a program simply because you interviewed for a position. Your top priority is to consider your own goals and personal preferences. Interviews are not only for the program to assess applicants, but also for you to get a feel for what your life will be like over the next year. However, you must ask yourself, "Would not having a residency be better than spending a potentially difficult year at this particular program that is not a fit for me?" If the answer is "yes," take that program out of consideration entirely.

> If you feel a residency program may not be ideal but will properly train you for your future plans, rank them. The last thing you want to do is not rank a program and be left scrambling. Despite some blogs from students stating they matched via the Scramble and were better off than if they'd matched with their 7th choice, the reality is that they are the <10% who match in the Scramble, and the odds are not in your favor.

Factors to consider when constructing your rank order list will likely be the same as you considered when deciding which programs to apply to initially. Only now you have additional information and insight gained during the interview process. Although ASHP-accredited programs follow the established guidelines, there is a variety in institutional philosophy and patient care, and educational and research experiences offered. By thoroughly investigating each program, you will be able to determine which program you feel is the best fit for your practice philosophy and career goals. Revisit those same criteria that you previously considered important (see Appendix B: Factors to Consider When Evaluating Individual Programs). However, this time you will have additional information and perhaps a lot more of your questions answered. Some additional thoughts that may be elucidated after your interviews:

- *Mission of the residency program*—Does it meet your career goals?
- *Opportunities in patient care, research, and/or teaching*—Do they meet your needs? Is the residency or fellowship program as advertised?
- *Geographic location*—Is there a particular area of the country that you find more desirable?
- *Type of institution*—Do you have a preference for academic versus nonacademic settings, large versus small, Veterans Affairs versus Public Health, which you did not have previously?
- *How did you feel during the interview*—Can you see yourself working there and integrating into the pharmacy team?
- *Interactions with RPDs and preceptors*—Will they meet your learning and mentoring needs? Does their teaching philosophy match what you are looking for?

 After interviews, it is not uncommon for your priorities to change. For example, you may start thinking, "Wow, the type of institution is not as important as I thought." Or, "Wow, I would prefer to be at an institution that offers teaching opportunities." As such, it's okay to feel overwhelmed and confused... just take some time to let your thoughts settle.

After you have considered all your variables, you can determine if a program does or does not fit your needs and will be on your rank order list. Additionally, these factors may give you assistance in determining your actual program rank order for submission. You may find a program that has everything you are looking for and is a perfect fit; thus, this would be at the top of your list. You may find other programs that may not offer one or two things you are looking for, but where you are a good fit and they assist in meeting your career goals, so these positions may fall further down on the list. Theoretically, if you did due diligence while screening for residency positions to submit applications to, most of the places you interviewed should be ranked.

As for how many programs to rank, this question goes back to how many programs you applied to or interviewed with (see Chapter 5: Formally Applying and Getting Ready for a Pharmacy Residency Interview). Sometimes this may be restricted by geographic location, resources, or time off from advanced pharmacy practice experiences (APPEs), as well as other considerations. There are no limits to the number of programs you can rank so you may rank each program that you interview with that you find meets your needs. Additionally, there are no guarantees that the likelihood of matching is increased if you rank more programs. The best way to increase your ability to match with a program is to be thorough in your assessment of the programs and apply to those that best fit your needs and rank them according to your level of interest. *Let us repeat*, you are best served by ranking programs based on your true level of interest. Depending on your relationship with the individuals you used as references, you may be able to ask for their advice to aid you in selecting your rank order as they may have completed one or more residencies themselves. Do not be afraid to ask for their opinion keeping in mind that their opinion is just that—their opinion—and it may not be right for you.

Submitting Your Rank Order

When the Match submission period opens, you may begin submitting your rank order selections as many times as you wish until the submission period is over. Be sure to submit your rank order well in advance of the deadline, as many applicants will be attempting to access the RMP system close to the deadline, and you want to make sure your rank order is submitted on time.

During this same time period, you may also withdraw your rank order up until the RMP submission period closes. If for any reason you have to withdraw your rank order list (or remove a program from the list) prior to the submission deadline, your ability to seek an unfilled position will not be affected after the release of Match results (during what is known as the Scramble), but keep in mind there is no guarantee that residency positions will be available during this time period.

> **Submit your rank order as soon as you have it settled.**

One of the editors once had two students within the same year. Mike was a solid student who secured seven interviews out of 18 applications he sent. After interviewing, he decided to rank all his choices despite having two that were out of the state and far from his family and girlfriend. Icarus was a great student who secured seven out of 10 applications he sent. After interviews, he ranked six programs but decreased it to three the night before the submission period ended since he felt confident that he would match with one of his top three choices based on his high grades/involvement, high rate of securing interviews, positive communication perceived from the RPD and preceptors during interviews, and his own reluctance to travel. Match Day arrives. Mike matched with his seventh choice, 12 hours away from home. Icarus did not match, went through the Scramble, and despite securing interviews still did not match. Mike spent a great year at his residency site, excelled, and became engaged (to a different girl) and is pursuing a fellowship, which he never would have pursued if not for the opportunities presented by his residency program. Icarus spent a year in community pharmacy and did not reapply the following year (for reasons described in Chapter 11: Congratulations and Encouragement). Moral of the story: Don't be like Icarus, be like Mike!

Algorithm

The matching process itself is relatively simple and does not require a complicated computer-based algorithm, but a computer is used to facilitate matching of applicants with program positions. The algorithm begins with tentative matches for each applicant's most preferred program, provided the most preferred program has an unfilled position. If the tentative match cannot be obtained with the applicant's most preferred program, the algorithm attempts to match the applicant with the next choice and continues until the applicant's rank order is exhausted. All matches are initially tentative, because once an applicant is matched for a position, another applicant could be preferred more by that program, removing the first applicant from that position.

MATCH DAY AND PLANNING FOR THE SCRAMBLE

After you have submitted your rank order, think about where you will be and how you will react when the Match results are released. Would you like to look up your Match results by yourself so you can gather your thoughts before you share your news with the world? Or is a Match Day party with other applicants more your style? Also, it is a good idea to mentally prepare ahead of time for matching with your ideal program, not matching at all, or matching somewhere in between. Once you have matched with your ideal program and have shared your exciting news with your family and friends, be sure to let your mentors and references know which lucky program gets to work with you next year. More than likely you have worked with these individuals as an intern, on advanced pharmacy practice experiences, or during research projects, and they want to see you do well, so keeping them apprised of your Match status is part of professional courtesy.

 Remember to ask your preceptor for Match Day off in case you do not match and have to scramble. Be prepared to make up those missed advanced pharmacy practice experience hours on extended days or weekends.

It is okay to share your news via Facebook® or Twitter®. However, refrain from stating, "I matched with my number one choice." Again, pharmacy is a small world and you don't want to make any enemies. Instead state, "I matched with the University of Tennessee. I am so excited…Rocky Top, here I come!" or "I matched with St. Anne's in Chicago… I am so pumped…Can't wait to start!" It will be more diplomatic and shows professionalism on your behalf.

Because residency positions are growing increasingly competitive, the application process does not stop with the release of the Match results. Prior to the release of the Match results, start thinking about those references that you would be able to contact because you feel they might be able to help you find an unfilled position during the Scramble period. If you did not match, do not despair, the application process continues with the Scramble, covered in the next chapter.

KEY LESSONS

- The Residency Matching Program is designed to match applicants and programs who are interested in each other.

- If you properly screened programs before submitting applications, programs with which you interviewed (except on rare occasions) should be ranked.

- It is essential that you choose your rank order based on your true preferences, not which program(s) you believe will rank you.

- Keep important dates like rank order submission deadlines in mind throughout the residency application process.

- Submit your rank order as soon as you have it settled to avoid any complications.

- Plan for your results on Match Day—either way.

REFERENCE

1. ASHP Residency Matching Program. Available at http://www.natmatch.com/ashprmp/. Accessed February 10, 2012.

CHAPTER 9

YOU DID NOT MATCH...TIME TO SCRAMBLE

Jehan Marino, PharmD, BCPP

Jessica Wine, PharmD

Note: If you did match, skip ahead to Chapter 10: You Matched.

You worked diligently over the past six months preparing for the residency application process and heeded all the advice this book offers (or maybe not); however, you received an e-mail that leaves you on the sidelines—you did not match. You may feel like you have been punched in the gut, are experiencing a nightmare, or are in disbelief—you may even cry. That's okay, since it means you are human and have feelings after all. To some of you, this may be the first major disappointment of your academic career. Unfortunately, not every applicant matches, but this is not the end of your career. In fact, each year, many residency applicants do not match (approximately 40%), and even some well-regarded programs do not match with their selected applicants (http://www.natmatch.com/ashprmp/).[1] You should not take this situation personally. Failure to match does not mean you are an unqualified or poor applicant, nor does it mean that the unmatched programs are undesirable. It is imperative to stay positive and not to get discouraged. The key is to focus and move on quickly to achieve your goal of securing a quality residency position. Remember, there may be another 1,500 students in the same position, all scrambling for one of the 100 to 200 remaining programs. You do not have the luxury of having a pity party as the remaining programs will fill up fast. You need to move deliberately but with great haste.

PRACTICAL STEPS TO TAKE

The following steps can be helpful in navigating through the Scramble process:

1. *Ask to take Match Day off*—As mentioned in previous chapters you should have done this prior to finding out the results of the Match. In the event that you do not match, this will allow you to quickly respond to the programs that are unmatched and to mentally prepare yourself for the Scramble. This is also a good time to contact your references letting them know that you did not match and that you will need them to resend letters to the new programs you identify.

2. *Obtain the "Scramble list"*—Through the Pharmacy Online Residency Centralized Application Service (PhORCAS), you will have access to the new dynamic post-Match list of all the residencies still available. Of note, unlike previous years, this list will be updated regularly as the positions get filled; therefore, you will not be left wondering and spending a lot of time and resources contacting a residency program director (RPD) who may have filled his or her remaining slots.

 Typically, applicants will know if they've matched prior to 9:00 a.m. The list of unmatched positions does not come out until about 12:00 p.m. Use this time wisely.

---

3. *Be open and flexible*—Being open to residency programs in different regions of the United States will increase your chances of securing a position; however, if you are restricted to a certain region or state, focus on the open positions listed in your specified area. Also, consider being open to different types of programs you were not initially interested in. For example, say you were set on doing a pediatric-focused postgraduate year-1 residency; however, your initial search did not locate any in your area. This may not be a bad thing. Keep in mind, most programs will try to accommodate an applicant's interest by either providing that rotation or recommending another nearby institution that will allow the resident to gain the experience in their area of interest.

4. *Be prompt and contact the RPD from your identified list of programs*— E-mailing the contact person of the residency program your

curriculum vitae (CV) and personal statement (PS) *and* following up with a phone call is strongly recommended. This shows the RPD that you are proactive and truly interested in pursuing their program. Make sure to stay professional and calm during all communications. Remember, the unmatched program is also eager to fill their position, so be patient!

 Be patient! Residency program directors may receive 100–200 e-mails/voice-mails within 24 hours.

---

5. *Request letters of recommendation to be sent to programs* — Most programs in the post-Match Scramble will require letters of recommendation to better assess you as an applicant since they may not have gotten to know you earlier in an on-site interview. Therefore, immediately forward the new contact information of your identified residencies to your references to ensure they will expeditiously submit additional positive letters of recommendation. Even if additional recommendations are not requested, it may be in your best interest to stand out as an applicant with strong letters of recommendation in your favor. If you did not update your references on your status, or if there is a chance they are unfamiliar with the Scramble timeline, you may wish to politely underline the importance of timeliness at this stage.

6. *Talk to your faculty preceptors or mentors* — Most likely, your professors or preceptors were in your shoes going through the same process at one point, so lean on them for support and advice. They also have relationships in the profession and have colleagues in different parts of the country and may give you guidance on leads to unfilled residency positions. Also, during the Scramble, some institutions or pharmacy programs gain funding for a new position, which can open up opportunities for those applicants that did not match initially. These programs may not be accredited (or may be in the accreditation process); however, it may give you more flexibility in your residency experience.

Questions You May Have During the Scramble

■ *"Do unmatched programs take applicants that did not apply to their programs the first time around?"*

The simple answer is yes! Residency programs are in a similar position as you in filling their empty position(s). Put your best foot forward and properly research the programs to show your interest in them as a potential post-Match applicant.

■ *"Should I contact a program that has an open slot if I previously applied or interviewed there?"*

Again, the answer is yes! The Match process is somewhat complicated, and you may have been a highly coveted applicant that did not make the cut-off. Some programs receive over 70 applicants for one to two positions and may not have the resources to interview all the applicants they want. Your selection for an interview represented that you were selected from a wide range of initial applicants and may have been considered high caliber, just not their first choice. Again, it is not personal. If you did interview at a particular site, you may have an advantage (unless you interviewed poorly). Do not let your ego get in the way, especially if you genuinely liked the program. Contact them and see what happens.

If You Don't Match in the Scramble

If after reading this chapter, and following all of the steps above, you still have not successfully secured a residency position, do not be deterred. According to ASHP, only 10% of unmatched residency applicants match during the Scramble.

Helpful Tips

We offer some helpful tips on how to proceed. First, take time to reassess your career goals. Do you still want to complete a residency? If the answer is yes, then we suggest the following:

■ Contact an RPD

- Speak with the programs you interviewed with and ask which area(s) of your application they feel you could improve on to make you a more viable applicant.

- Expand your CV
  - With the year ahead, gain experience and/or add to your CV (especially in the RPD-identified areas of improvement) to make you stand out the second time around.
  - Consider enrolling in a course or certificate program (e.g., medication therapy management, consultant, immunizations) to help address clinical domain deficiencies.
  - Pursue volunteer opportunities that will allow you to work with a specific patient population and/or enhance your communication skills. While the RPD may not be able to measure your improvement, following these steps will demonstrate that you had the insight to recognize a shortcoming, put together a plan to address it, and execute the plan. Successfully completing this process can help make a very compelling case for your candidacy.
- Find a job
  - You may consider applying to the same practice setting as your future residency position. Most of these jobs would be *per diem* and give you a "leg up" compared to residency applicants who just obtained their licenses. You would also learn to navigate their computer system and logistical support. If you do take this route and secure a job, remember to treat this job as a one-year interview.
- Get involved in scholarly activity
  - Keep in contact with your previous faculty and preceptors to find out if there is an opportunity to participate in a new research project or assist with any of their ongoing research.
  - Be open to assisting in co-authoring a manuscript with a faculty or preceptor to gain writing experience and be recognized by your peers. Working *per diem* in a pharmacy setting will provide you with the free time to complete some scholarly activity.
- Be active in the profession
  - Get involved in health fairs or screenings—this may be an opportunity to network with other pharmacists and RPDs.

- Assist colleagues by participating in the peer-review process for manuscripts. Speak to your professors or preceptors to get started.

SUMMARY

While working to enhance and improve your CV, keep in mind that the residency search starts up again in the fall. Be proactive! Follow the previously discussed steps. Make sure to broaden your search and keep your options open. Your goal is to secure a large number of interviews so that after you narrow down your viable options, you still have a decent number to rank.

DR. WINE'S STORY OF STRUGGLE AND SUCCESS: DOING IT RIGHT THE SECOND TIME AROUND

I was extremely disappointed in not matching the first time around. I was the type of student who from the first day of pharmacy school planned on completing a residency after graduation. When I did not match (even through the Scramble) I thought, "What could I have done wrong?" I had worked hard in all my classes/APPEs and received excellent grades (i.e., Rho Chi) in pharmacy school. Being left unmatched, I went through an emotional rollercoaster of depression, disappointment, and anger, finally leading to acceptance and excitement to reapply in the upcoming year as an outstanding residency applicant. I took the year to gain professional experience and learn more about myself both personally and professionally. To gain professional experience post-Match, I was offered an opportunity from one of my preceptors, Dr. Caballero, to be lead author on a review article.[2] Not only did writing the review article keep me motivated to move forward in my career, it also gave me opportunities to complete peer reviews of other upcoming manuscripts. Additionally, Dr. Caballero took the time to advise me on how to approach the interview process the second time around (e.g., reapplying, expanding my search to more programs, interviewing tips, evaluating my CV/PS).

Before sending out my application, Dr. Caballero served as my second set of eyes, evaluating my CV and PS for errors. Furthermore, he prepared me with mock interview questions so I became more adept at thinking on my feet during the real interview. I quickly recognized the rookie mistakes I had made the first time around when I had not asked for any advice; I had only applied to three programs, thinking all would grant me interviews and be rankable for the Match. I was wrong on all counts.

After numerous consultations with my preceptor to make sure I was ready for the second go-around, in early November, I began contacting RPDs via e-mail, introducing myself and explaining my situation of not matching the first time and my immense interest in reaching my goal this time. I described my pending publication and desire to complete a pharmacy practice residency. I also visited some local residency programs on-site prior to submitting my application to introduce myself in person (since I was unable to attend the Midyear Clinical Meeting) and obtain more information about each program. By the time residency applications were due, I had added to my CV a publication that was accepted and soon to be published in a well-regarded, Medline-indexed pharmacy journal, making me stand out from applicants who were just graduating. I applied to nine programs (instead of three programs the previous year) and received requests for on-site interviews from eight. I initially found preceptors wary of the "blank space" in my career. However, after meeting with me, the programs appeared to admire my persistence and were intrigued by my dedication to complete a residency and achieve my career goals. When asked to explain, I described the activities I had completed during the year that set me apart from other applicants still completing pharmacy school. I was able to rank five programs and matched with one of my top picks. The moral of the story: DO NOT GIVE UP! Put your best foot forward and be humbled by life's little hiccups.

KEY LESSONS

- Do not give up or get discouraged if you did not match the first time around...persistence often pays off.

- Ask for advice from past preceptors and faculty members for moral support and to assist in ways to improve your curriculum vitae, personal statement, and/or interviewing style.

- Act quickly to ensure a future position.

- Be open and flexible to new programs and areas that were not your initial choice, but still align with your career goals.

References

1.   ASHP Residency Matching Program. Available at http://www.natmatch. com/ashprmp/. Accessed March 30, 2012.

2.   Wine JN, Sanda C, Caballero J. Effects of quetiapine on sleep in nonpsychiatric and psychiatric conditions. *Ann Pharmacother.* 2009;43(4):707-713.

CHAPTER 10

YOU MATCHED

Matthew Seamon, PharmD, JD

Congratulations! You matched! You might feel like this is the end of a long and arduous journey, but it is not. It certainly is an important milestone and an earned accomplishment, but it is not the checkered flag. It is only the beginning of the next chapter in your professional career. There is important work to be done and time now becomes an issue.

OUT WITH THE OLD

Match results become available in mid-to-late March. Many graduations are not until late May or even June. Residencies typically commence the first week of July. Accordingly, as a graduating student you will likely have a number of outstanding responsibilities to deal with. These may range from finishing advanced pharmacy practice experiences (APPEs) and completing research papers to such mundane tasks as returning library books or paying parking tickets to the university. Do not overlook these responsibilities as your goal is to start with a fresh mind. Such lapses can delay a release of your grades (or diploma) which most institutions will ask for prior to commencing your residency. (See **Table 10-1**.)

Table 10-1. Top Ten Things to Do—Out with the Old, In with the New

OUT WITH THE OLD

- ❑ Successfully complete all remaining advanced pharmacy practice experiences and earmark time for studying for licensing exams.
- ❑ Send thank-you e-mails to your dean, professors, mentors, and colleagues, as applicable, sharing your news and providing new contact information when available.
- ❑ Call a family meeting to discuss your expectations for the upcoming year and listen to their concerns and worries.
- ❑ Confirm that you have met all of your academic and university related responsibilities, as not to delay graduation or licensing.

❏   Close out living arrangements such as ensuring security deposits are returned, utilities are turned off, and lease obligations are met.

❏   Determine moving plans, such as using professional movers versus a U-Haul® type of vehicle and identifying people to help with moving.

❏   Schedule maintenance of your car (e.g., changing oil, air tire pressure).

❏   Take some time to contemplate your success. Consider things that worked for you in pharmacy school and things that you would have done differently (learning from your past).

❏   Complete any outstanding professional tasks such as manuscript submission, projects, and giving notice to your current employer.

❏   Schedule a celebratory dinner with friends and family.

IN WITH THE NEW

❏   Contact the board of pharmacy and initiate pharmacy licensure application.

❏   Identify study materials for the North American Pharmacist Licensure Examination (NAPLEX®) and state law exams.

❏   Establish personal and residency goals for the upcoming year.

❏   Contact your new program director and identify any pressing responsibilites. Gather all necessary contact information for your residency (both e-mail and telephone) so you always have access to appropriate personnel.

❏   Finalize living arrangements, open bank account with direct deposit, contact your loan holder to discuss repayment options, and request additional credit from your current credit card company.

❏   Purchase new lab coat and update wardrobe as necessary. Consider new climates and need for lighter, more comfortable clothing (e.g., linen and cotton) or heavy warmer clothing (e.g., down and wool).

❏   Establish primary route to work, learn traffic patterns and public transportation options, develop alternate routes in case of traffic or closures, register for an electronic toll collection system (e.g., E-ZPass®) to improve driving time, and estimate travel time to work.

❏   Evaluate benefits at work such as dental, healthcare, and prescription drug coverage. Find a new local physician and pharmacy as needed. Schedule initial appointments and get new prescriptions, if necessary.

❏   Take some time to reset and refresh. Garner excitement, enthusiasm, loyalty, and discipline for your program. Purchase new supplies if needed such as computers, pens, notebooks, and drug information resources. Activate or update home Internet service as applicable.

❏   Schedule a meet-and-greet with your new colleagues. This will show your initiative, collegiality, and friendliness. Always maintain professionalism, limit access to alcohol, and present your best self.

Meeting with Family and Friends

Consider sitting down with your loved ones and having a formal discussion of the pressures and challenges ahead. These may include the pressures to succeed, extended working shifts and schedules, conflicts with new personalities on the job, personal adjustments, new living conditions and environments, and the possible realization that a job may not always be as glamorous as advertised. Even though you are a Doctor of Pharmacy, residency stipends are not full salaries, and unanticipated financial constraints may be felt. This is a time of profound growth and change. Do not underestimate the road ahead. You have prepared your entire academic career for what you are about to embark upon. Having the support of family and friends will make the transition easier and provide the support that may be necessary during the ensuing year. A residency is filled with highs and lows and pressures abound. Also, consider that the road ahead may provide unaccustomed stresses. Coping mechanisms become essential to success as a resident and happiness as an individual.

Self-Evaluation

Now is also a good opportunity to reflect and do some professional introspection. Do you want to be the first person at work in the morning and the last to leave in the evening, or are you satisfied to simply check off the residency box on your curriculum vitae (CV) and collect a paycheck? You may be better suited to further cultivating your strengths in a residency by focusing projects, assignments, and rotations on areas in which you are strong and well versed. On the contrary, you may benefit more by trying to address your weaknesses as the challenges provide motivation to stay inspired and ultimately make you a better, more well-rounded practitioner. Do you work better alone or in a group? Understanding and identifying some of these characteristics will only enhance your professional development and job satisfaction.

If you have remaining APPEs, now is the time to finish strong and not tail off. Understand that in a few short months you will be a licensed pharmacist, meaning a heightened level of responsibility and expectation. Yes, as a resident there is still education to be obtained and a preceptor to report to, but as a resident pharmacist, you will be viewed by your peers with a high level of collegiality and expectation. Seek to learn as much as you can on your remaining APPEs. Arrive early and leave late (you really should be doing this already). It will give you the opportunity to learn the facts and equipment that you may have been shying away from. Start or finish any assignments you've neglected. This will be your schedule for the year and it is a great opportunity to acclimate yourself to the upcoming responsibilities.

Especially for individuals that match locally, this is an additional opportunity to demonstrate your real worth to your colleagues. Wrap up any projects you have outstanding, both personally and professionally. Come day one of your residency or fellowship, the change in scenario and newfound responsibilities are going to require your complete devotion and attention. Any lingering issues will only serve as a distraction.

 Once residency begins, it will be extremely difficult to complete and submit that manuscript you were working on as a student.

Now is also a good opportunity to wrap up research, or publish a paper that might have stalled as you focused on getting a residency. As the competitive landscape of pharmacy evolves, publications will be an important differentiating characteristic looked upon by future employers. This is a good opportunity to work again with that preceptor who inspired you. Consider contacting your preceptor and letting them know that you matched and are interested in publishing the paper you had worked on. Seek to submit the paper before the residency begins, while the information is still relatively fresh, and before the new set of responsibilities begins. You have worked this hard already; now see things to completion. It will also give you important experience and confidence that will aid your residency. Alternatively, this may be a good opportunity to approach an individual at your residency and seek early collaboration on a project. Having an ally at your new workforce and a kick start will only help. If you are remaining local, it may be a good idea to meet with your future residency program director (RPD) and start developing your research idea/project (be proactive). In fact, the research project may be an extension of work you have already been doing.

A colleague of mine once had a student who asked to work on a research study. After presenting the abstract and poster at a national pharmacy conference, the student kept delaying finishing the project and submitting the manuscript. The day after the Match and securing a residency position, she e-mailed him stating she no longer wanted to complete the project. A year later, this student was looking for a postgraduate year-2 (PGY-2) residency and submitted her CV to several programs. One of the RPDs she interviewed with knew that earlier preceptor and asked about the presented abstract. Afterward, she contacted the preceptor stating she had a very tough decision between two "phenomenal" applicants. The former preceptor was tactful and forwarded the original e-mail in which the student withdrew from the project. Needless to say, the decision became quite simple for the RPD. There are many, many other stories like this. Moral of the story: *finish what you start!* (And pharmacy is a small world after all—but if you have been reading, you should know that by now.)

Conduct a resource assessment and evaluation of your technological needs. Is the computer you have sufficient to meet the job's needs? Do you need to upgrade or purchase a smartphone? Are your drug information sources sufficient in scope and ease to meet your professional responsibilities? The quality and access to resources vary greatly among programs. It is appropriate to ask what is available so you do not pay for information that may be freely available. Additionally, as a member of the program you may qualify for special rates on smartphone plans, or other resources, so inquire.

If you plan on relocating, there are a number of important considerations. You must find a new place to live. Asking the current residents about places to live and recommendations is helpful. Some institutions even have formal relocation programs to help. Walk a fine line, however. Although it is appropriate to ask for recommendations, do not appear overly needy. Searching for a place to live online is a great resource in today's environment.

 Do not be afraid to ask the landlord for a discount stating you will be a pharmacy resident that will be professional, will not trash the place (since you will be working a lot) and more importantly, have a *stable* income where paying rent every month on time will not be a problem. You have no idea how many landlords would love to have a tenant like yourself.

Finances

Financial issues and constraints may pose new concerns for you at this time. Inquire about student loans and deferment opportunities available with your lender. Again, now is the time to deal with these issues—not on the residency clock. You may need to open a new bank account, especially if you are relocating. Remember many employers utilize some form of direct deposit, where your paycheck is directly deposited into your account. This is often preferred by your employer and should be viewed as a beneficial convenience for you as well. Some banks may even offer free checking and banking with direct deposit. Some institutions may be associated with credit unions. Also, check to see which automated teller machines (ATMs) are most readily available at the hospital and around your future home. This will save you money on ATM charges that can add up (remember, you'll still be a resident). The key is the more research you do on your employer, the more benefit you may derive.

Now is a good time to consult a financial planner (or other resource) and start budgeting. As this will be the first pharmacist paycheck of your career, unforeseen tax consequences may arise and spending can quickly exceed earnings. Different states have different tax requirements and a qualified accountant will serve you well. For example, working and living in a major city may have additional taxation, and thus living outside the city limit may ease that burden. Budgeting will help you achieve your goals. This may range from meeting your monthly expenses to beginning to contribute to a retirement plan or even a college savings plan if you have children. The key is to begin to develop good financial habits that will follow you throughout your career.

A large portion of you will have high interest rate/subsidized loan issues and the reality that you may not be able to defer loan payments during postgraduate training. Therefore, it is imperative that you consult with your lender to determine how much you will be paying per month. Some institutions offer these services for free so take advantage of them.

Insurance matters are another consideration at this point, especially pharmacy malpractice insurance. There are a number of carriers and a simple phone call may demonstrate that malpractice insurance is less expensive and easier to obtain than one would think. Malpractice insurance is strongly recommended, especially for a novice pharmacist and is inexpensive (less than $200 per year) to obtain (https://www.personal-plans.com/ashp/welcome.do). Car insurance may need to be changed if you are moving and own a car. Some companies offer discounts based on occupation (i.e., pharmacist) or bundling. You may even start investigating life insurance plans, as rates are lower and more readily available when you are young.

Perhaps your car needs a good tune-up to last you a year (or two) or you may need to buy a newer car. Again, calculate your finances before you decide to splurge on a car you cannot afford. However, make sure your transportation is reliable and will not be a distraction or an excuse for tardiness or absenteeism. Alternately, you may be moving to a city (e.g., Chicago, New York) where public transportation is reliable and you may not need to have a car. As a result, consider selling your car or leaving it behind to save money on parking spaces, gasoline, and insurance (e.g., larger cities most likely have higher car insurance premiums than smaller cities). After calculating expenses, one of my students was able to save over $200 per month on using public transportation instead of owning a car.

Bidding Farewell

Now is also a good time to extend the personal and professional thanks to the people that helped you achieve this milestone. An e-mail or handwritten thank-you note to a dean, faculty member, or preceptor that helped you along the way will be viewed favorably and goes a long way. Stopping by in person to extend your gratitude is even better. It does not have to be a long visit; five minutes is more than enough for a sincere visit. Saying goodbye to your classmates, friends, and former life may be a difficult proposition to many and the pressures of being a licensed and responsible professional are new. Nevertheless, you should approach these situations with confidence and excitement and the realization you are prepared for the challenge and successes.

IN WITH THE NEW

As the Match triggers a number of closing responsibilities, it also triggers a number of important new considerations. Start off by e-mailing your future RPD and colleagues and express your excitement to work with them. Ask if there is anything specific you can do at this time. Inquire about required paperwork and human resource materials. You may get together with other future residents (if programs accept several residents) and gauge your similar interest. Remember you will be working long hours with them for a year (or more). For example, during a residency in Texas, a group of new residents found a mutual interest for football. As a result, the residents, their spouses, and some pharmacy and other doctoral students formed a flag football team which played on Friday nights. After a long week, they would gather to have some fun and decompress. Even if some of the residents did not play, they would show up for support. Afterward, they would go have dinner and a good time.

Setting a Good Example at Work

Follow up promptly on all requests from your program. It demonstrates dedication and commitment. It will also work to expedite and facilitate the hiring and starting. Some programs are well established and experienced, and paperwork may already be in the mail. Burgeoning programs may still be a bit disordered and your attention and timeliness will be appreciated. The goal is a seamless first day, and avoiding pitfalls. You do want to get paid on time, right? Identify key staff members who will help make your start easier and approach them with respect and appreciation, as these attributes go a long way. Support staff (e.g., administrative assistants, technicians) can make your life very easy or very unpleasant—avoid being condescending and demanding. Key staff often have their finger on the pulse of an institution as well as the politics within. They can also assist you with minor or logistical issues that do not merit the attention of your RPD or preceptors. You never know when you may need a favor.

Start reading all the policies and procedures available regarding your position and your institution. Employee handbooks are a great source of information. Consider scheduling a telephone or in-person meeting with a human resource employee, if needed.

Realize the residency year goes fast. Start thinking ahead. What practice settings are you interested in pursuing after your residency? What is your area of research and interest? Although you may not have definitive answers to these questions at this point, understand that some will, and they may have a competitive advantage accordingly. If you can sit down early on in your residency planning and address these issues, it will only serve to kick start your year and demonstrate to your colleagues your focus and attention. Are you planning on pursuing a PGY-2 or fellowship? If so, where? In what specialty? Are you seeking to gain employment back at a hospital where you completed an APPE or at your residency site? Answers to these questions will help foster development and allow you to schedule the best 12 months possible. October arrives quickly and for some of you, you will begin the entire process over again in searching for a PGY-2 or fellowship (or maybe even your first job as a pharmacist).

PHARMACIST LICENSURE

On top of everything else, you must begin concentrating on your board exams and state pharmacist licensure application. As soon as you match you should contact your respective state board of pharmacy for an application. Typically there is a pharmacy component, such as the North American Pharmacist Licensure Examination (NAPLEX®), and a law component, such as the Multistate Pharmacy Jurisprudence Examination (MPJE®). Treat both sections equally and importantly. Research the application requirements to avoid any unexpected delays, as some nuances exist between states. Some states may have requirements that prove problematic for certain individuals and those will have to be communicated to your RPD. For example, Florida forbids licensure as a pharmacist to individuals convicted of healthcare fraud. Also, some states require more intern hours than others for licensure. Consult your state licensing board for specific requirements and bars from licensure.

Consider getting licensed in the state in which you and/or your family currently reside or other states in which you might even consider relocating after residency. Although the application fees may seem expensive, the exam scores can easily be transferred at this point, the study materials are still fresh, and it helps establish a contingency plan.

CONTINGENCY PLANS

By participating in the Match, you agree to report to the residency program. However, you may not ever start or even finish the residency. Therefore, having a contingency plan is a reasonable contemplation. This plan should include financial reserves, demographic considerations (where to live), occupational considerations (i.e., back-up job), and personal values and goals.

Reasons you may not start a residency could be personal, health-related, or financial. Some programs may require you to be licensed after a certain period of time and you may fail to get licensed and be forced out. Additionally, institutions may merge or downsize, RPDs may be terminated from employment or leave of their own accord, programs may lose funding, or natural disasters (e.g., hurricanes, tornados) can occur. There have been instances where residency funding has been pulled and a matched applicant was left without a residency. At this time, ASHP is working on how to address these issues. However, if this occurs, you may want to consult a lawyer to discuss your options.

Some residencies are a disappointment, and some residents are a disappointment. There may exist a time before completion of the residency that a mutual ending is sought. While this is highly discouraged, it happens. However, be aware that leaving a residency may greatly impact your ability to secure another residency (and certain types of employment) at a later time. Hopefully, all of the interviewing and time spent to date will minimize this risk.

A component of a contingency plan may include getting licensed in another state. Also, keeping or finding part-time employment elsewhere can provide fall-back financial resources and opportunities upon completing a residency. However, the rigor and schedule of your residency may simply not allow this. Keep in mind, also, that any part-time job during your residency will distract you from your primary responsibilities and ability to perform at your best in your program, which should be your ultimate goal. Additionally, some residencies may have a schedule where having a part-time job will be close to impossible and you will need your rest whenever you can get it. Have you been considering going back to school for a masters degree? Now may be a good time to consider and research this option. Your program may even contribute to the cost. You may not have the time for such an endeavor but simply having the information will help ease the burden in case something unexpected happens.

Having a cash reserve is highly recommended. You may be starting a program with little or no money, but now is the time to start building this reserve. Although you may have sufficient resources for one or two months of living expenses saved, you will want to start and save for more. Car repairs are costly, renewals for pharmacy licensures come quick, insurances often come in lump bills, and even the cost of replacing a wet cell phone can feel catastrophic without the proper reserve. Also, one should carefully assess the need for building a strong credit line with the risk of over-extending credit at this point. *Seek to continue to live and spend as you did a student.* The time is short-lived, and you do not want to develop bad habits or get off on the wrong foot, which may impact your career in unimaginable ways or for an extended duration.

 You may not receive any income for two to four weeks, depending on how payroll distributes payments. Make sure you have enough financial resources for that initial period.

VACATION

Plan a vacation—even if it's a "stay-cation." Look for three to four days (preferably a week) where you can go and decompress before you start your residency. Some move a week or two earlier and spend time exploring the city and doing all the "fun stuff." Believe it or not, you may finish a residency in New York and never have the time to visit the Metropolitan Opera, or leave Knoxville without ever enjoying a football weekend while listening to "Rocky Top." Make sure you take time to enjoy your life— you'll finish your residency, work, and perhaps marry and have kids someday (and maybe even watch your kids have children of their own before you know it).

SUMMARY

Matching with a program deserves a huge sigh of relief and a long pause for excitement; but remember, there is work to be done and this is really just the start of another chapter. Finish up strong with the old and embrace the new. In front of you is the opportunity you spoke about during your residency or fellowship interview and spent so much time writing about in your personal statement. You are a pharmacist and will officially be in the position to help people and improve lives. Soon enough you will have your residency certificate in hand and your next set of responsibilities and pressures ahead. So prepare yourself for an intense year of residency, but remember to stop every once in a while to see how much you have accomplished and enjoy the ride.

 KEY LESSONS

- Develop and reinforce good habits immediately. Work hard, be courteous to others, and be knowledgeable of your expectations. The times they are a-changing!

- Conduct a self-evaluation of your personal and professional goals as soon as your Match results are posted.

- Understand the financial situation you will be in. Continue to live modestly, as you did as a student.

- Get licensed quickly. Apply early, test early, pass! Don't get caught by any surprises. Your livelihood and reputation may be indelibly marked.

- Consider developing a contingency plan in case your residency ends unexpectedly.

- All of your hard work and dedication has paid off. Reflect on your accomplishments and prepare yourself for the pressures and challenges ahead. Celebrate your Match!

CHAPTER 11

CONGRATULATIONS AND ENCOURAGEMENT

Joshua Caballero, PharmD, BCPP

Kevin A. Clauson, PharmD

Sandra Benavides, PharmD

This book has covered a lot of information that will assist you in securing interviews and more importantly, in securing a residency or fellowship. Recurrent themes throughout the book have focused on being organized, proactive, and detail-oriented. Most importantly, though, is remaining true to yourself. The guidance in this book puts you in the best possible position to succeed in your goal of securing postgraduate training. If you do succeed in securing a residency or fellowship...Congratulations! However, even if you do not secure a position after all your efforts, life does not end. You will have several months before you have the opportunity to start the process all over again as a more experienced applicant.

 If you do not succeed in securing a residency or fellowship the first time, do not get discouraged—take some time to heal your pride, but reapply!

If history is any indicator, the vast majority of you who do not secure a position the first time around will not seek a residency or fellowship in subsequent years. From over 30 combined years in academia, the editors have only seen a handful of students go through the interview process a second time. After you start your new job as a community or staff pharmacist, you can fabricate a million excuses to not pursue one. We have heard them all, including:

- Things happen for a reason; I guess it's not for me.
- If they did not want me the first time, why would they want me now?

- I will not or cannot sacrifice my salary and comforts of a job that currently pays close to (or more than) six figures.

- I want to get a few more years of "experience" before reapplying to make me a better applicant.

- I am now married and cannot afford it.

- I want to have children before reapplying because (fill in the blank).

- I am burned-out from school, so I will take a break/rest for a year or two and reapply.

- Any other excuse that translates to "I am bitter that I did not get a residency the first time around."

- Any other excuse that translates to "I was so severely embarrassed/humiliated by the outcome the first time around that I cannot bear to go through it again."

When looking at some of our nation's icons, it is sometimes those that persevered and overcame failures that have the most success including Henry Ford, Walt Disney, and Bill Gates. Therefore, if completing a residency is something you really and truly desire, *you will find a way*. In your life, you probably have succeeded in most things you have done; do not allow one setback to change your track record. Remember to stay true to yourself, focus, work hard at becoming a better applicant, and reapply. In conclusion, may all your efforts come to fruition in moving our profession forward!

Preparing Your Curriculum Vitae: Format and Headings

Personal Information (TOP OF FIRST PAGE)

John Alexander Lemus

1452 NW 15th Avenue
Miami, FL 33125
Phone: 555-555-5555
E-mail: john.a.lemus@network.com

Professional Objective

Optional, but it is generally left off the curriculum vitae (CV). Some state, "To secure a residency that..." but professional objectives can do more harm than good as they state the obvious, appear unoriginal, and take up space. Your intentions of applying to a residency or fellowship program are apparent, and besides, your personal statement (PS) will expand on this.

Education and Experience

This includes all professional degrees earned such as BA, BS, MS, and PharmD. This section needs to include the school name/location where degree was obtained and the dates of attendance. Most human resource departments will confirm degrees and may ask for a performance assessment (e.g., transcripts). Of note, there are some students that add grade point average (GPA) after their degrees (e.g., GPA: 3.53). However, it is not a necessity. For example:

2008–present   Doctor of Pharmacy, University of Tennessee Health Science Center; Memphis, Tennessee (anticipated graduation date: May 2012)

2004–2008   Bachelor's of Arts in Psychology, University of Florida; Gainesville, Florida

Licensure and Certification

Include your pharmacy intern license(s) (or other licenses you may have) information including state(s) and dates issued. Also, include any certification(s) you have received such as tobacco cessation training, immunization training, and teaching certificates. For example:

2011–2013	American Heart Association Basic Cardiac Life Support Certification
April 2010	Bone Density Screening Training
October 2009	APhA Immunization Delivery Certificate
October 2009	Florida Intern Pharmacist License 2984578 (expires October 2013)

Honors and Awards

This can go as high up on your CV as following the licensure and certification section or later in the CV. It can also be omitted entirely if you do not have any. For example:

May 2011	First Place Florida Society of Health-System Pharmacists Clinical Skills Competition
2010–2012	Rho Chi Honor Society, Gamma Theta Chapter
2010–2012	Phi Lambda Sigma Honor Society, Omega Chapter

Professional Work Experience

This typically includes all internships and research positions held. Your supervisor's name in each position should also be listed; however, avoid including contact information such as an address, e-mail, or phone number. You should include a brief description of responsibilities. Dates of employment should be on the left margin, so that they stand out easily. For example:

2010-2012	Pharmacy Intern, Prescription Drugs Pharmacy; Miami Beach, FL
	Supervisor: Richard S. Finkel, PharmD
	Role: Obtained verbal telephone orders from prescribers, assembled pharmacy policies and procedures for on-site immunization program, assisted pharmacists in counseling patients, created software to manage pharmacy technician scheduling

2009–2012   Research Assistant, Nova Southeastern University; Fort Lauderdale, FL

Supervisor: Dexter Brunson, PharmD, BCPS

Project title: Text messaging to improve adherence in patients with type 2 diabetes

Role: Collected background information for the study, assisted with Institutional Review Board (IRB) preparation, enrolled patients, data entry to Excel, editing of abstract/poster preparation and presentation

Advanced Pharmacy Practice Experiences

List each experience with the name of the advanced pharmacy practice experience (APPE) and location (including site, city/state, and preceptor). Additionally, have two to three sentences or four to six bullets describing the experience as stated in Chapter 2: Developing Your Curriculum Vitae and Personal Statement. Dates of experiences should be on the left margin. For example:

March 2012   Internal Medicine I

Memorial Southern Hospital; Miami, Florida

Preceptor: Robert Batard, PharmD, BCPS

Responsibilities:

- Rounded with medical team
- Recommended drug therapy
- Provided pharmacokinetic monitoring (e.g., vancomycin)
- Presentation: Linezolid for vancomycin resistant *Enterococcus*
- Drug utilization review: Daptomycin
- Assisted preceptor in reviewing a manuscript submitted to *American Journal of Health-System Pharmacy*

 If you reviewed a manuscript with a preceptor, *do not* state the name of the article or even the topic as you may unknowingly expose the blinded review process.

Introductory Pharmacy Practice Experiences

Similar to APPEs, list each experience with the name of the introductory pharmacy practice experience (IPPE) and location (including site, city/state, and preceptor). Additionally, have two to three sentences describing the experience as stated in Chapter 2: Developing Your Curriculum Vitae and Personal Statement. Dates of experiences should be on the left margin. For example:

October 2009 – McGyver's Compounding Pharmacy; Coral
April 2010   Springs, Florida

                 Preceptor: Jennifer Bradley, PharmD

                 ■ Filled prescriptions

                 ■ Compounded and dispensed medications
                    to patients

                 ■ Processed transfer of prescriptions

Research Experience

List each experience with the name of the study, location (healthcare setting and/or university), and primary advisor. You may add two to three bullets stating your role and if you submitted/presented a poster or manuscript. For example:

2010–2011   The relationship between medication adherence and
                cognition in patients with HIV, Nova Southeastern
                University; Fort Lauderdale, FL

                Prinicipal Investigator: Paul Stern, PharmD

                ■ Role: Collected background information for the
                   study, assisted with IRB preparation, data entry to
                   Excel

                ■ Submitted abstract to ASHP Midyear Clinical
                   Meeting (pending decision)

PUBLICATIONS

Use standard PubMed formatting. For example:

2012   **Lemus JA**, Benavides S, Caballero J, Clauson KA. Using text
           messaging to improve adherence and health outcomes in patients
           with type 2 diabetes. *Am J Health-Syst Pharm.* 2012;69(5):400-404.

2011   **Lemus JA**, Caballero J, Benavides S, Clauson KA. The use of text messaging to improve adherence in type 2 diabetes. *Am J Pharm Educ.* 2011;74(Article 8):3. [abstract]

PRESENTATIONS

Keep your APPE and professional presentations separate. Core items include author(s), presentation title, audience(s), specific site, and city/state along with month and year. You can also include the type of presentation in parentheses (e.g., poster, platform presentation) to enhance clarity. For example:

Professional Meeting Presentations and Posters

July 2011   **Lemus JA**, Caballero J, Benavides S, Clauson KA. The use of text messaging to improve adherence in type 2 diabetes. Presented at the American Association of Colleges of Pharmacy Annual Meeting, San Antonio, TX, July 2011. [poster]

- Assisted with IRB submission
- Designed database
- Assisted with recruiting and consenting patients
- Obtained blood samples (e.g., point-of-care tests)
- Assisted with data entry and abstract development
- Edited poster presentation

 If you presented at a pharmacy conference, the audience does not need to be defined. However, if it is a conference that someone reviewing your curriculum vitae is not familiar with, then consider defining the audience.

IPPE and APPE Presentations

March 2012   Appropriate use of antidepressants in the elderly

- Presented at Memorial Southern Hospital; Miami, FL (1 hr)

- Audience: Pharmacists, physicians, and medical students
- Objective: Discuss the initial dosing and proper titration of antidepressant therapy
- Secondary objective: Discuss significant drug interactions, common side effects, and patient counseling

---

Any topic you have presented and included in your curriculum vitae is fair game to the interviewer, so know your presentation(s) inside and out!

Membership and Service to Professional Organizations

List your memberships to all local, state, and national organizations. Remember to specify the specific chapter name. Dates are unnecessary unless you have held specific positions in professional organizations. It is important to provide a description of what you contributed under service roles as stating the name of the role does not tell the person reading your CV what you did. Being president of an association does not indicate leadership by virtue of the name *president*. Cite examples of your accomplishments that highlight your impact. If you carried an initiative forward in your role as secretary or treasurer, again, it is important to highlight this. For example:

2010–present   Phi Lambda Sigma Honor Society, Omega Chapter

Vice-President, 2010–2011

- Planned and organized various leadership workshops specific for students
- Ensured that logistics for all planned events were well-organized

Secretary, 2009–2010

- Arranged room reservations and recorded meeting minutes
- Offered tutorial sessions for students
- Assisted in professional and fundraising events

2009–present   Alliance of Students Against Poverty

Ω   President, 2009–2010

- Established an organization that focused on the eradication of poverty in the Philippines
- Helped plan a conference for university students from Florida to raise awareness on the struggle against poverty
- Organized Hunger Banquet with Oxfam to support the fight against global hunger
- Coordinated fundraising and community events

Community Service

List community service activities and any volunteer events that you participated in. Stick with only those completed during pharmacy school. For example:

June 2011   Argentina Medical Mission; Mar del Plata, Los Cardales, Argentina

- Interprofessional team (e.g., pharmacists, physicians, dentists, students) assessed, evaluated, and treated underserved patients
- Provided therapeutic drug recommendations and alternatives
- Counseled patients on medications

April 2011   Southern Spring Wellness Day, Nova Southeastern University; Fort Lauderdale, Florida

- Operation Medicine Cabinet: Worked with a pharmacist and the county sheriff in the documentation and handling of medications
- Properly disposed patients' unused medications, especially controlled substances

March 2010   Tenth Annual ASSIST Health Fair; Bell Glades, Florida

- Planned booth's activity with pharmacy advisor

- Completed training on US Preventive Services Task Force (USPSTF) guidelines for bone density screening and use of dual energy x-ray absorptiometry (DEXA) scanner
- Counseled patients on proper lifestyle modifications

 If you were interviewed for a newspaper or television piece regarding any healthcare-related event, you may place it under a heading of Media Appearances.

Media Appearances

January 2010   Tome Control De Su Peso; Hialeah, Florida

- 20-minute interview in Spanish
- Interviewed for television educational piece regarding obesity

FACTORS TO CONSIDER WHEN EVALUATING INDIVIDUAL PROGRAMS

- Type of training experience (postgraduate year-1 [PGY-1], post-graduate year-2 [PGY-2], fellowship)
- Institution characteristics
  - Geographical location
  - Type of institution (teaching, community, etc.)
  - Size of institution
  - Number of sites (inpatient, ambulatory care, etc.)
  - Patient populations/services provided (geriatrics, pediatrics, transplant, etc.)
  - Travel requirements
- Stipend/funding
  - Cost of living
  - Public transportation
  - Financial/resource support to travel to conferences to present
- Staffing or service requirement
  - Location of staffing
  - Type of staffing (order entry, clinical services, on-call, etc.)
  - Frequency of staffing
  - Coworkers when staffing
- Number of resident/fellow positions
  - PGY-1
  - PGY-2 (which specialties)
  - Fellows (which specialties)

- Residency program director (RPD) and preceptors
  - Credentials and years of experience
  - Qualifications and training of the preceptors
  - Additional certifications (BCPS, AAHIVE, etc.)

 If you can't tell the difference with pharmacy credentials between CDE and CIA, you probably want to review this resource on the topic: http://www.pharmacycredentialing.org/ccp/Files/CCPWhitePaper2010.pdf.

- Rotations offered
  - Schedule format and flexibility
  - Basic/required rotations
  - Elective/optional rotations
  - Unique possibilities for new rotations
  - Offsite or collaborative experiences with other institutions
  - Experiences in your particular area(s) of interest
  - Flexibility in changing rotations if your area of interest changes

---

 If toward the end of your residency, you have secured a future position (e.g., clinical job, postgraduate year-2, fellowship), you may want to ask if you can change your rotation to one that will better prepare you for the next phase of your career.

- Current residents
  - Behaviors and attitudes
  - Opinions and experiences regarding preceptors, rotations, and program as a whole
  - Reported pros and cons
  - Suggestions for improvements
  - Would they choose this residency if they were given the choice to do it all over again
  - Future plans (what do they plan to do after they finish, did their residency experience play a role in that decision)
- History of the program
  - How many years since inception/number of previous graduates

- Where did previous graduates obtain employment/how many residents have been retained
- Major changes to requirements, directorship, or programs structure recently implemented or planned

■ Professional opportunities
- Networking
- Collaboration
- Involvement in professional organizations/committees
- Teaching certificate and/or academic experiences
- Publication and other scholarship opportunities

POTENTIAL QUESTIONS ASKED DURING RESIDENCY INTERVIEWS

■ Personality related
- What qualities do you possess that would make you a good resident?
- What are your worst qualities?
- What are your short-term (e.g., 2–5 years) and long-term goals (e.g., 10 years)?
- What three words would your best friend use to describe you?
- Do you prefer to work individually or as part of a group?
- What has been the most difficult situation you have faced, and how did you handle it?
- If you had to critique your own performance, where could you improve?
- What do you think is your greatest strength?

- Tell me about a time you failed and what you learned from it.
- Describe a situation in your professional career where you felt *stressed* or encountered *conflict*.
- What do you like to do for fun?
- How do you handle stress?
- Why are you the best candidate for this program?

■ Professionally related

- Why did you attend pharmacy school?
- Why do you want to do a residency?
- Why are you interested in our program? *versus* Why did you choose to interview for this program?
- Where do you see yourself after completing the residency?
- What areas of pharmacy most interest you?
- Are you considering a postgraduate year-2 (PGY-2) residency or fellowship?
- Describe how pharmacy practice is changing and what you see as being relevant for the future.
- What is the single most important facet of interpersonal communication?
- What can you offer our program that other applicants cannot?
- Would you consider yourself to be innovative? Why or why not?
- Are you an introvert or an extrovert and how does that impact your approach to direct patient care?
- How do you envision the role of the pharmacist in the patient-centered medical home?
- How has technology and automation negatively impacted the profession?
- Given (example scenario), how would you handle the situation?

- Describe your time-management skills.

- Describe a leadership role that you had.

- How do you define Medication Therapy Management?

■ Experiential

- What is your definition of a clinical pharmacist?

- What was your favorite advanced pharmacy practice experience (APPE) and why?

- How could you have improved your least favorite APPE?

- Describe your favorite or most memorable patient.

- Describe your most memorable experiences from APPEs.

- If I were to ask preceptor X to describe you, what words would he or she use?

- Who was your favorite preceptor and why?

- Describe or discuss the most interesting medical journal article you have recently read.

- Why are critical thinking skills an important quality in a clinician?

- Describe a conflict with a preceptor or attending physician and how it was resolved.

- Describe the most significant contribution you made to a patient's care this past year.

- Do you think the Health Insurance Portability and Accountability Act is accomplishing what it was intended to?

Source: Originally published in Mancuso C, Paloucek F. Understanding and preparing for pharmacy practice residency interviews. *Am J Health-Syst Pharm*. 2004;61(16):1686-1689. ©2004, American Society of Health-System Pharmacists, Inc. All rights reserved. Adapted with permission.

MIDYEAR CLINICAL MEETING RESIDENCY SHOWCASE FLOOR PLAN EXAMPLE

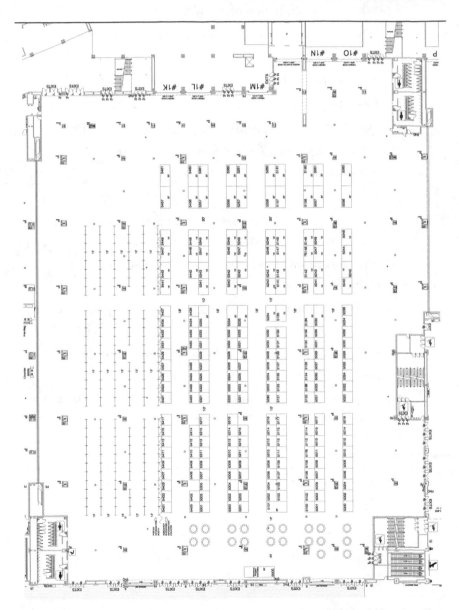

Source: Residency showcase and personnel placement service floor plans. Available at http://fp37.a2zinc.net/clients/fpashp/2011MidYear/public/fp.aspx?EventID=8&MapID=23&ContactID=0. Accessed February 14, 2012.

MIDYEAR CLINICAL MEETING PERSONNEL PLACEMENT SERVICE FLOOR PLAN EXAMPLE

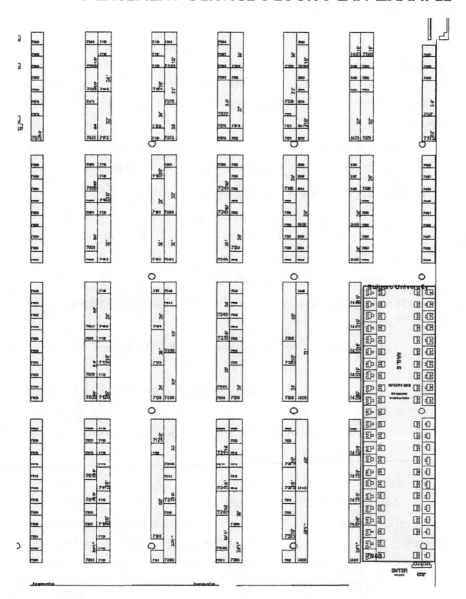

Source: Residency showcase and personnel placement service floor plans. Available at http://fp37.a2zinc.net/clients/fpashp/2011MidYear/public/fp.aspx?EventID=8&MapID=23&ContactID=0. Accessed February 14, 2012.

QUESTIONS TO ASK AND AVOID WHEN INTERVIEWING

Asking good questions can show you are prepared, interested in an institution's residency or fellowship program, and eager about the opportunities there if you match. Good questions you might ask include the following:

- What are some positions that your former residents have taken and that current residents are seeking after completing the residency?
- What choices are available for the elective months?
- Which electronic medical record system, if any, does your hospital use? What challenges have been encountered with this system?
- How would you describe the relationship between pharmacy, medicine, and nursing departments?
- What is your teaching philosophy for your residents versus your students?
- I noticed that you have an affiliation with University X. What teaching opportunities are available?
- I noticed that Children's Hospital Y is in your vicinity. Is it possible to do a rotation there?
- (For non-accredited programs or fellowships) Does your program have any follow-up procedures after the interview?
- (For non-accredited programs or fellowships) What is your policy or timeline for offering positions to applicants?

Inappropriate questions imply you may have something better to do, or that you are sweating the small stuff. Some of these details are important (e.g., vacation, work hours); however, they can be asked *after* you get the residency. Common inappropriate questions asked include the following:

- How many hours do we staff?

- How many vacation/sick days do we get?

- How early in the day do we start?

- What time do we normally stop?

- Do we have to carry a pager and be "on call"? If so, how often is that?

Some students are getting bad advice about looking for a residency that has *no* staffing hours. Staffing is a vital component of a residency providing experiences that will make you a better pharmacist. These opportunities include the following:

1. Learning the drug distribution system, computer software, and pharmacy logistics

2. Learning the cognitive processes involved in the drug approval process, knowledge of drug formulations and administrations, and circumstances requiring specially prepared formulations

3. Making decisions in a short amount of time as a staff pharmacist (understanding the stress)

4. Learning prescribing patterns of physicians (good or bad)

5. Sharpening your order entry/verification skills

6. Knowing *you* are the last person to verify a medication before it is dispensed

---